Revision Facial Plastic Surgery: Correcting Bad Results

Editors
PAUL S. NASSIF
JULIA L. KEROLUS

FACIAL PLASTIC SURGERY CLINICS OF NORTH AMERICA

www.facialplastic.theclinics.com

Consulting Editor
J. REGAN THOMAS

November 2019 • Volume 27 • Number 4

ELSEVIER

1600 John F. Kennedy Boulevard • Suite 1800 • Philadelphia, Pennsylvania, 19103-2899

http://www.theclinics.com

FACIAL PLASTIC SURGERY CLINICS OF NORTH AMERICA Volume 27, Number 4
November 2019 ISSN 1064-7406, ISBN-13: 978-0-323-71038-1

Editor: Jessica McCool
Developmental Editor: Laura Kavanaugh

Facial Plastic Surgery Clinics of North America (ISSN 1064-7406) is published quarterly by Elsevier Inc., 360 Park Avenue South, New York, NY 10010-1710. Months of issue are February, May, August, and November. Business and Editorial Offices: 1600 John F. Kennedy Blvd., Suite 1800, Philadelphia, PA 19103-2899. Periodicals postage paid at New York, NY, and additional mailing offices. Subscription prices are $408.00 per year (US individuals), $659.00 per year (US institutions), $454.00 per year (Canadian individuals), $820.00 per year (Canadian institutions), $535.00 per year (foreign individuals), $820.00 per year (foreign institutions), $100.00 per year (US students), and $255.00 per year (foreign students). Foreign air speed delivery is included in all *Clinics* subscription prices. All prices are subject to change without notice. POSTMASTER: Send address changes to *Facial Plastic Surgery Clinics*, Elsevier Health Sciences Division, Subscription Customer Service, 3251 Riverport Lane, Maryland Heights, MO 63043. **Customer service: 1-800-654-2452 (US and Canada); 1-314-447-8871 (outside US and Canada); Fax: 314-447-8029; E-mail: journalscustomerservice-usa@elsevier.com (for print support); journalsonline support-usa@elsevier.com (for online support).**

Reprints. For copies of 100 or more of articles in this publication, please contact the Commercial Reprints Department, Elsevier Inc., 360 Park Avenue South, New York, NY 10010-1710. Tel.: 212-633-3874; Fax: 212-633-3820; E-mail: reprints@elsevier.com.

Facial Plastic Surgery Clinics of North America is covered in *MEDLINE/PubMed* (*Index Medicus*).

Contributors

CONSULTING EDITOR

J. REGAN THOMAS, MD, FACS
Professor, Facial Plastic and Reconstructive
Surgery, Department of Otolaryngology–Head
and Neck Surgery, Northwestern University
Feinberg School of Medicine, Chicago, Illinois,
USA

EDITORS

JULIA L. KEROLUS, MD
Clinical Assistant Professor, Division of Facial
Plastic and Reconstructive Surgery,
Department of Otolaryngology–Head and Neck
Surgery, University of Illinois College of
Medicine, Chicago, Illinois, USA

PAUL S. NASSIF, MD, FACS
Director, Nassif MD, Inc and Associates,
Beverly Hills, California, USA; Assistant Clinical
Professor, Department of Otolaryngology–
Head and Neck Surgery, Keck School of
Medicine of USC, Los Angeles, California, USA

AUTHORS

MARTIN J. CITARDI, MD
Department of Otorhinolaryngology–Head and
Neck Surgery, McGovern Medical School, The
University of Texas Health Science Center at
Houston, Houston, Texas, USA

ROBERT T. CRISTEL, MD
Division of Facial Plastic and Reconstructive
Surgery, Department of Otolaryngology–Head
and Neck Surgery, The University of Illinois at
Chicago, Chicago, Illinois, USA

RICHARD E. DAVIS, MD
Voluntary Professor of Facial Plastic and
Reconstructive Surgery and Facial Plastic and
Reconstructive Surgery Fellowship Director,
The Division of Facial Plastic and
Reconstructive Surgery, Department of
Otolaryngology, University of Miami Miller
School of Medicine, Miami, Florida, USA;
Director, The Center for Facial Restoration,
Miramar, Florida, USA

SEAN W. DELANEY, MD
Huntington Ear Nose Throat Head & Neck
Specialists (Private Practice), Pasadena,
California, USA

NEIL A. GORDON, MD, FACS
Founder and CEO, New England Surgical
Center, The Retreat at Split Rock, Wilton,
Connecticut, USA; Director, Head and Neck
Aesthetic Surgery, Coordinator, Facial Plastic
and Reconstructive Surgery, Assistant Clinical
Professor, Department of Surgery, Section of
Otolaryngology, Yale School of Medicine, New
Haven, Connecticut, USA

AMAR GUPTA, MD
Department of Otolaryngology–Head and Neck
Surgery, NYU School of Medicine, New York,
New York, USA

JOHN BRYAN HOLDS, MD, FACS
Ophthalmic Plastic and Cosmetic Surgery,
Inc., Des Peres, Missouri, USA; Departments of
Ophthalmology and Otolaryngology–Head and
Neck Surgery, Saint Louis University School of
Medicine, St. Louis, Missouri, USA

ARI J. HYMAN, MD
Private Practice, Facial Plastic and
Reconstructive Surgery, Encino, California,
USA

LESLIE E. IRVINE, MD
Santa Barbara Plastic Surgery Center, Santa Barbara, California, USA

WEE TIN K. KAO, MD
Fellow, Division of Facial Plastic and Reconstructive Surgery, Department of Otolaryngology, University of Miami Miller School of Medicine, Miami, Florida, USA

ANDREW J. KAUFMAN, MD, FACP
Director, The Center for Dermatology Care, Thousand Oaks, California, USA; Clinical Associate Professor of Medicine, Keck School of Medicine of USC, Los Angeles, California, USA

JULIA L. KEROLUS, MD
Clinical Assistant Professor, Division of Facial Plastic and Reconstructive Surgery, Department of Otolaryngology–Head and Neck Surgery, University of Illinois College of Medicine, Chicago, Illinois, USA

SARAH KHAYAT, MD
Division of Facial Plastic and Reconstructive Surgery, Department of Otolaryngology–Head and Neck Surgery, The University of Illinois at Chicago, Chicago, Illinois, USA

RUSSELL W.H. KRIDEL, MD
Facial Plastic Surgery Associates (Private Practice), Division of Facial Plastic Surgery, Department of Otorhinolaryngology–Head and Neck Surgery, McGovern Medical School, Clinical Professor, The University of Texas Health Science Center, Houston, Texas, USA

WENDY W. LEE, MD, MS
Bascom Palmer Eye Institute, University of Miami Miller School of Medicine, Miami, Florida, USA

GRACE LEE PENG, MD, FACS
Facial Plastic and Reconstructive Surgery, Beverly Hills, California, USA

ROBI N. MAAMARI, MD
Ophthalmic Plastic and Cosmetic Surgery, Inc., Des Peres, Missouri, USA; John F. Hardesty, MD Department of Ophthalmology and Visual Sciences, Washington University School of Medicine, St Louis, Missouri, USA

GUY G. MASSRY, MD
Beverly Hills Ophthalmic Plastic and Reconstructive Surgery, Beverly Hills, California, USA; Orbital Center, Cedars Sinai Medical Center, Department of Ophthalmology, Division of Oculoplastic Surgery, Keck School of Medicine of USC, University of Southern California, Los Angeles, California, USA

PHILIP J. MILLER, MD
Department of Otolaryngology–Head and Neck Surgery, NYU School of Medicine, New York, New York, USA

PAUL S. NASSIF, MD, FACS
Director, Nassif MD, Inc and Associates, Beverly Hills, California, USA; Assistant Clinical Professor, Department of Otolaryngology–Head and Neck Surgery, Keck School of Medicine of USC, Los Angeles, California, USA

ABDUL NASSIMIZADEH, MBChB, BMedSci, MRCS
University Hospital Birmingham, Birmingham, United Kingdom

MOHAMMAD NASSIMIZADEH, MBChB, BMedSci, MRCS
University Hospital Birmingham, Birmingham, United Kingdom

JAYAKAR V. NAYAK, MD, PhD
Division of Rhinology–Endoscopic Skull Base Surgery, Department of Otolaryngology–Head and Neck Surgery, Stanford University School of Medicine, Stanford, California, USA

THOMAS GERALD O'DANIEL, MD, FACS, EMBA
Founder and Director O'Daniel Plastic Surgery Studios, Founder Louisville Surgery Center, Clinical Assistant Professor, Department of Plastic Surgery, University of Louisville, Louisville, Kentucky, USA

BORIS PASKHOVER, MD
Assistant Professor, Department of Otolaryngology–Head and Neck Surgery, Rutgers New Jersey Medical School, Newark, New Jersey, USA; Division Chief, Facial Plastics and Reconstructive Surgery, St. Barnabas Medical Center, Robert Wood

Johnson Barnabas Health, Livingston, New Jersey, USA

AMY PATEL, MD
Beverly Hills Ophthalmic Plastic and Reconstructive Surgery, Beverly Hills, California, USA; Orbital Center, Cedars Sinai Medical Center, Los Angeles, California, USA

ANDREW J. RONG, MD
Bascom Palmer Eye Institute, University of Miami Miller School of Medicine, Miami, Florida, USA

PATRICK STAROPOLI, MD
Bascom Palmer Eye Institute, University of Miami Miller School of Medicine, Miami, Florida, USA

JASON TALMADGE, MD
Department of Otolaryngology, Medical College of Wisconsin, Kenosha, Wisconsin, USA

DEAN M. TORIUMI, MD
Division of Facial Plastic and Reconstructive Surgery, Department of Otolaryngology–Head and Neck Surgery, The University of Illinois at Chicago, Chicago, Illinois, USA

JACOB I. TOWER, MD
Resident, Department of Surgery, Section of Otolaryngology, Yale School of Medicine, New Haven, Connecticut, USA

ANN Q. TRAN, MD
Bascom Palmer Eye Institute, University of Miami Miller School of Medicine, Miami, Florida, USA

YAO WANG, MD
Beverly Hills Ophthalmic Plastic and Reconstructive Surgery, Beverly Hills, California, USA; Orbital Center, Cedars Sinai Medical Center, Los Angeles, California, USA

JINLI WU, PA-C
Donald B. Yoo, M.D., Inc, Facial Plastic and Reconstructive Surgery, Beverly Hills, California, USA

WILLIAM YAO, MD
Department of Otolaryngology, Medical College of Wisconsin, Kenosha, Wisconsin, USA

DONALD B. YOO, MD
Donald B. Yoo, M.D., Inc, Facial Plastic and Reconstructive Surgery, Beverly Hills, California, USA; Division of Plastic and Reconstructive Surgery, Department of Otolaryngology–Head and Neck Surgery, University of Southern California, Los Angeles, California, USA; Division of Facial Plastic and Reconstructive Surgery, Department of Otolaryngology–Head and Neck Surgery, University of California, Los Angeles, Los Angeles, California, USA

Contents

Postblepharoplasty lower eyelid retraction is challenging and multifactorial and may occur after transcutaneous lower eyelid surgery. Surgical correction is difficult and unpredictable. Patient psyche is often negatively affected. This combination of events can limit patient satisfaction, so significant preoperative counseling to educate patients and modulate expectations is critical. The combination of midface lifting, implantation of a posterior lamellar spacer graft, and canthal suspension (standard surgery) has led to variable degrees of functional and aesthetic improvement. This article reviews the typical presentation, outlines the steps of standard surgery, and touches on other modalities of treatment that may improve patient satisfaction.

Fat grafting is effectively used in the lower eyelid and periorbital area for rejuvenation of the aging face. Several complications may occur with fat grafting, including volume undercorrection or overcorrection, contour irregularities, prolonged bruising and swelling, infection, granulomas and inflammation, and vascular embolization with visual loss or stroke. In many cases, complications can be effectively treated, although permanent and serious injury can occur. Appropriate surgical techniques help to prevent most of these complications. An understanding of how and why complications of fat grafting of the lower eyelid occur aids in the avoidance and treatment of these complications.

Iatrogenic septal perforation is a complication of nasal surgery. Small or posterior perforations cause few symptoms, and need only conservative treatment. Larger and anterior perforations contribute to nasal airflow disturbances and external nasal deformities. When considering surgical candidacy, one should consider the severity of symptoms, location and size of the perforation, and need for revsional rhinoplasty. We repair perforations using intranasal mucosal advancement flaps augmented by an interposition connective tissue graft. Septal perforation repairs are tedious and technically challenging. We review key points to minimize unintended perforation formation following nasal surgery.

Overzealous reduction during rhinoplasty may result in manifold functional as well as aesthetic injuries to the nose and is a prevailing antecedent of revision rhinoplasty.

Although challenges for the revision rhinoplasty surgeon abound, careful assessment of the anatomic deficiencies of the nose, accurate evaluation and management of a patient's expectations, and precise planning and execution of surgical technique serve to facilitate a successful result. Contemporary techniques for correction of the over-resected nose are discussed, with special attention directed toward costal cartilage grafting and diced cartilage fascia techniques.

Empty nose syndrome (ENS) is a controversial condition associated with disruption of nasal airflow caused by excessive loss of turbinate tissue. ENS arises after total or near-total inferior turbinate resection. Patients present with intense fixation on the perception of nasal obstruction. Diagnostic tools to assess for empty nose syndrome include a validated patient questionnaire and the office cotton test. Treatment involves topical moisturization, behavioral/psychiatric assessment/treatment, and surgical reconstruction. Current data show promising long-term efficacy after surgical intervention. Postprocedural ENS is best prevented by minimizing inferior and middle turbinate tissue loss.

The pinched nasal tip deformity often results as sequelae of prior nasal surgery. Conventional tip surgery techniques that overemphasize tip narrowing often deform the lateral crura and weaken support for the alar margin. The pinched nasal tip is characterized by the demarcation between the nasal tip and the alar lobule, isolating the tip from the surrounding nasal subunits. Lateral crural strut grafts with or without repositioning offer the surgeon a powerful maneuver that can help correct this functional and aesthetic deformity and restore a natural appearance to the nasal tip.

The cephalic trim technique is a popular maneuver that often leads to tip deformities, most notably postsurgical alar retraction (PSAR). We advocate using the external rhinoplasty approach to correct PSAR by (1) releasing and repositioning the retracted alar margin, (2) strengthening and immobilizing the central tip complex using a septal extension graft, (3) suspending and longitudinally tightening the mobilized lateral crural remnant by adjusting crural length to match the sidewall span, and (4) providing direct skeletal support to the repositioned alar margin using articulated alar rim grafts. Using this structural treatment paradigm, we have corrected severe PSAR in the preponderance of secondary rhinoplasty cases.

As the number of patients seeking surgical and nonsurgical rhinoplasty continues to increase, the risk of nasal skin compromise after surgery also has risen. Vascular insult to the nasal skin envelope can lead to permanent disfigurement that is nearly impossible to correct. Tissue loss often requires major reconstruction that yields suboptimal cosmetic results. This article discusses prevention, early recognition, and effective treatment that aim to mitigate skin necrosis and the resulting soft tissue destruction.

An ideal scar is flat, thin, and color matched to the surrounding skin. Incision planning, skin closure, and postoperative care are vital to create an inconspicuous scar. Depressed, hypertrophic, and keloid scars each pose unique challenges to the facial plastic surgeon. Several surgical and nonsurgical options exist in the treatment of scars. Appropriate treatment is based on scar location, quality, and size as well as patient history, preferences, and expectations. This article discusses techniques for prevention and treatment options for unsightly and hypertrophic scars.

Complications of rhytidectomy are well known, yet often preventable. A thorough preoperative history and physical along with realistic patient expectations provide the surgeon and patient with insight into potential complications and postoperative management. Understanding of surgical pitfalls and avoidance are crucial in beginning to manage facelift complications. Possible complications of facelift techniques should not discourage surgeons from pursuing a particular technique as the majority of complications are temporary. Though, a strong patient-physician relationship is critical when complications occur. Complications may be frustrating for both the patient and surgeon, yet are overwhelmingly temporary and manageable without surgical intervention.

This article provides facial plastic surgeons with the insight to avoid and address common pitfalls in neck procedures. Many aesthetic issues are created from overtreatment or undertreatment of components of the neck. Using the platysma muscle as the divide, ease of access to superficial anatomy leads to overtreatment problems, whereas difficulty of access to deeper structures leads to undertreatment problems and to overall imbalances. Strategies to accurately assess and treat all structures of the neck proportionally can be used to both avoid and treat any neck aesthetic issues. The advent of minimally invasive techniques has resulted in new complications.

Soft tissue fillers continue to gain popularity in addressing volume loss and changes associated with facial aging. The rare but devastating complication from iatrogenic vascular occlusion can result in irreversible vision loss. This article discusses the complications of vision loss associated with fillers and reviews applicable treatment techniques and prevention methods.

This article discusses complications that may occur after procedures on the lips, specifically focusing on injectable fillers. Evidence-based guidelines and suggested methods to manage these complications are presented in a systematic format.

Andrew J. Kaufman

To avoid complications or bad results following reconstruction of skin cancer defects, there are several factors that can be incorporated into the design and execution of repairs. These techniques not only decrease the need to correct bad results, they improve the final aesthetic and functional outcome. So although one surgeon might focus on standard corrective treatments, another might use elements of flap design and implementation that will decrease the need for such corrective procedures. We discuss 4 useful reconstructive repairs and delineate the properties of design and execution that help to ensure success and avoid bad results.

FACIAL PLASTIC SURGERY CLINICS OF NORTH AMERICA

SERIES OF RELATED INTEREST

Clinics in Plastic Surgery
https://www.plasticsurgery.theclinics.com/
Otolaryngologic Clinics
https://www.oto.theclinics.com/

THE CLINICS ARE AVAILABLE ONLINE!
Access your subscription at:
www.theclinics.com

Foreword
Revision Facial Plastic Surgery: Correcting Bad Results

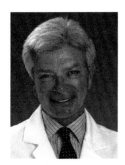

J. Regan Thomas, MD, FACS
Consulting Editor

All facial plastic surgery procedures and treatment modalities have potentially unintended outcomes, possible poor results, or complications. These issues should be minimized through proper preoperative planning, patient selection, and careful technique. However, even in the experience of well-trained and appropriately careful surgeons, complications can and do occur. Planning for correction of these unexpected and unfortunate situations should be part of the expertise and patient management methodology for all facial plastic and reconstructive surgeons' skill sets and patient care approaches. Although dealing with treatment complications can be challenging for both the surgeon, and indeed, the patient, it is imperative that proper and timely treatment approaches be recognized and appropriately utilized.

The Guest Editors, Dr Paul Nassif and Dr Julia Kerolus, have organized and selected an experienced group of authors to explore and discuss a wide spectrum of possible complications that may confront the reader as a facial plastic surgeon in this issue of *Facial Plastic Surgery Clinics of North America*. They have utilized the insights of surgeons from a variety of training backgrounds to explore an in-depth discussion of dealing with a wide variety of treatment challenges potentially presenting following aesthetic procedures. A goal of this issue is not only to describe appropriate treatment approaches for this variety of possible complications and poor result scenarios but also to discuss key elements of avoiding those outcomes for the initial treatment procedures.

Drs Nassif and Kerolus, through their carefully selected and experienced contributing authors, have created a useful and valuable reference for dealing with a variety of challenging but unfortunately inevitable aesthetic treatment outcomes and situations. Topics covered include surgical as well as popular injectable treatment modalities in an organized and systematic discussion that will prove to be relevant to today's treatment environment. It is my hope, as Consulting Editor, that this issue will provide the reader with innovative and clinically beneficial information that can be adopted as part of their expert care routine.

J. Regan Thomas, MD, FACS
Facial Plastic and Reconstructive Surgery
Department of Otolaryngology Head and
Neck Surgery
Northwestern University School of Medicine
675 North Saint Clair Street
Suite 15-200
Chicago, IL 60611, USA

E-mail address:
jreganthomas@gmail.com

Facial Plast Surg Clin N Am 27 (2019) xiii
https://doi.org/10.1016/j.fsc.2019.07.016
1064-7406/19/© 2019 Published by Elsevier Inc.

facialplastic.theclinics.com

Preface
Correcting Bad Results in Facial Plastic Surgery

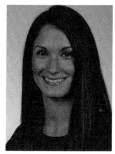 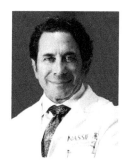

Julia L. Kerolus, MD   Paul S. Nassif, MD, FACS
Editors

Aesthetic procedures of the face and neck are increasing in popularity with emergence of innovative techniques and a shift in the social stigma of plastic surgery. With this rise, we are seeing an onslaught of patients with poor results or significant complications following cosmetic operations. Although knowledge of potential risks in aesthetic surgery is abundant, comprehensive information on management of these complications is lacking.

This issue of *Facial Plastic Surgery Clinics of North America* addresses the most common and feared complications in aesthetic facial surgery. It provides a framework for first-class management of aesthetic complications with articles authored by leading experts in the fields of facial plastic surgery, oculofacial plastic surgery, dermatologic surgery, and skull base surgery, each with a specialized niche for revision aesthetic and functional surgery.

We present a stepwise approach to treatment of periorbital, nasal, and facial deformity and functional sequelae following surgery, fat grafting, and dermal filler injection.

We would like to thank all of those who have contributed to this work. We have learned so much from assembling this issue, and our hope is that you find this collection useful in the management of your patients.

Julia L. Kerolus, MD
Division of Facial Plastic and
Reconstructive Surgery
Department of Otolaryngology–
Head and Neck Surgery
University of Illinois at Chicago-
College of Medicine
1855 W Taylor Street, Suite 2.42 (MC 648)
Chicago, IL 60612, USA

Paul S. Nassif, MD, FACS
Nassif MD, Inc and Associates
120 South Spalding Drive, Suite 301
Beverly Hills, CA 90212, USA

Department of Otolaryngology–
Head and Neck Surgery
University of Southern California
Keck School of Medicine
Los Angeles, CA 90033, USA

E-mail addresses:
julia.kerolus@gmail.com (J.L. Kerolus)
drnassif@drpaulnassif.com (P.S. Nassif)

Facial Plast Surg Clin N Am 27 (2019) xv
https://doi.org/10.1016/j.fsc.2019.07.015
1064-7406/19/© 2019 Published by Elsevier Inc.

Management of Postblepharoplasty Lower Eyelid Retraction

Amy Patel, MD[a,b], Yao Wang, MD[a,b], Guy G. Massry, MD[a,b,c],*

KEYWORDS

- Blepharoplasty • Lower eyelid retraction • Lower eyelid malposition • Lower eyelid ectropion
- Eyelid scar • Eyelid laxity • Eyelid volume

KEY POINTS

- Postblepharoplasty lower eyelid retraction (PBLER) is a challenging and multifactorial problem that primarily occurs after transcutaneous lower eyelid blepharoplasty.
- Identifying eyelid and periorbital deficits that underlie this eyelid malposition is critical to successful treatment.
- A more contemporary understanding of how volume loss, eyelid/cheek topography, and orbicularis deficit contribute to PBLER offers additional insights into the problem and other potential modalities of intervention.
- Surgical success depends on patient education, modulating expectations, sound surgical technique, and detailed attention to postoperative care.
- The psychological impacts of this complication are enormous, and patients require significant time and attention by physician and staff.

INTRODUCTION

Postblepharoplasty lower eyelid retraction (PBLER) is a multifactorial eyelid malposition that often leads to functional impairment, significant aesthetic deficit, and psychological trauma.[1,2] Its surgical correction is technically difficult, and lasting surgical outcomes require specialized training, a unique skill set, and the ability to manage postoperative tissue biology, including tissue contraction and wound healing. Clearly, this is a daunting task that should only be undertaken by those who will commit the time and energy necessary to allow the best and most consistent and reliable results

from this procedure. In the view of the senior author (GGM), who manages these patients routinely, assuming the responsibility of these patients can be physically, mentally, and psychologically stressful for both patient and surgeon. It is critical to keep this in mind when deciding to intervene in these cases because a good outcome only occurs when the patient is happy, and attaining this end is often difficult.

Traditional thought regarding the etiologic factors of PBLER is that it is related to transcutaneous (open-approach) surgery (reported in as high as 6%–20% of these cases)[3] and that it is associated

Disclosures: Dr G. Massry received royalties from Elsevier, Springer, and Quality Medical Publishers. The other authors have nothing to disclose.
[a] Beverly Hills Ophthalmic Plastic and Reconstructive Surgery, 150 North Robertson Boulevard #314, Beverly Hills, CA 90211, USA; [b] Orbital Center, Cedars Sinai Medical Center, Los Angeles, CA, USA; [c] Department of Ophthalmology, Division of Oculoplastic Surgery, Keck School of Medicine, University of Southern California, Los Angeles, CA, USA
* Corresponding author. Beverly Hills Ophthalmic Plastic and Reconstructive Surgery, 150 North Robertson Boulevard #314, Beverly Hills, CA 90211.
E-mail address: gmassry@drmassry.com

Facial Plast Surg Clin N Am 27 (2019) 425–434
https://doi.org/10.1016/j.fsc.2019.07.014
1064-7406/19/© 2019 Elsevier Inc. All rights reserved.

with 3 principal deficits: (1) unaddressed eyelid laxity, (2) anterior lamellar (skin or muscle) shortage, and (3) middle lamellar (orbital septal) scar.[4–7] Webster and colleagues[6] were the first to recommend canthal suspension (CS) as a preventative measure for PBLER after transcutaneous surgery. Since then, CS (whether a canthoplasty or a canthopexy) has become a mainstay in open-approach lower blepharoplasty and most assuredly has, to a degree, reduced the incidence of PBLER.[8–12] Until the 1980s, surgical correction of PBLER typically involved skin grafting, scar lysis as needed, and CS. Unacceptable scarring from skin grafts led to the development of an alternative means of adding skin to the lower eyelids, that being the recruitment of skin from below via trans-eyelid midface lifting.[1,4,7,13,14] In addition to skin recruitment, posterior lamellar spacer grafts were added to address the middle lamellar scar[14–17] and an open CS to support and secure the lower eyelid.[12,18–20] For the purposes of this article, this combination of midface lifting, spacer grafts, and CS (MSC) will be referred to as standard surgery. After MSC, the lower eyelid is typically put on stretch with some variant of tarsorrhaphy for the first 1 to 2 weeks postoperatively to help prevent wound contracture and maintain lower eyelid position.[1,13,17] Although many modifications of this approach have been reported, the initial descriptions by Shorr and colleagues of the modification known as the Madame Butterfly procedure are really the fuel that fed the engine of transeyelid midface lifting for correction of PBLER as it is known today.[1,13,17,21] The problem with this surgery is that, although it has consistently led to variable degrees of improvement in form and function, patient satisfaction has never formally been studied in an evidence-based manner.

In data gathered by the senior author (GGM; unpublished), patient satisfaction (40% by direct questioning) is significantly lower than surgeon satisfaction (80% by blinded assessment of patient photographs of outcome).[22] The authors believe surgeon satisfaction is high because lower eyelid position typically improves (surgeon's goal). However, patients must be heard and it is common for patients who have had MSC to complain of (1) an abnormal canthal appearance, (2) a shortened horizontal eyelid aperture, (3) hollowed lower lids, and (4) an ill-defined canthal and eyelid discomfort.[1] Number 4 is a real problem because corrective surgery may change form and structure; however, it is very hard to correct a feeling or sensation, especially when it is so difficult to describe. This led the senior author to study MSC outcomes in depth.[21] The findings will be described, and suggestions of alternative

paradigms that may simplify surgical intervention and recovery, and improve patient satisfaction, are suggested. However, the focus of this article is detailing the typical presentation of patients with PBLER and reviewing the steps and pearls of MSC.

PREOPERATIVE EVALUATION

Patients presenting with PBLER have a wide spectrum of findings, which will dictate the appropriate intervention. As stated, traditional thought with this deficit is that it is related to anterior lamellar shortage, a middle lamellar scar, and unaddressed eyelid laxity.[4–7] In line with this, the standard surgical intervention since the 1980s has been MSC. One of the authors (GGM) has studied patients with PBLER in detail and has identified that orbicularis weakness, a negative vector globe/midface morphology (prominent eye or negative vector eyelid), and a volume-depleted inferior orbit/lower eyelid are common findings in patients with PBLER that are unaddressed by standard surgery.[21] Also, as stated in a presentation at the annual American Society of Ophthalmic Plastic and Reconstructive Surgery scientific symposia in 2013,[22] the same author (GGM) demonstrated that patient satisfaction with MSC was significantly less that surgeon satisfaction (40% vs 80%). Why this discrepancy? It is possible that performing standard surgery on all patients, which has been the accepted standard, is a flawed approach?[1] Can alternative treatments, based on other findings not addressed by standard surgery, narrow the gap between patient and surgeon satisfaction?[1] These are excellent questions, which the authors continue to evaluate.

Although standard surgery is appropriate in many patients, when the findings suggest a primary deficit in volume, or topographic disparity of the globe and midface, filler injections are often enough and have yielded high patient satisfaction (Fig. 1).[1] Also, when orbicularis weakness predominates, performing orbicularis sparing or preserving surgery has shown to be beneficial and again has yielded high patient satisfaction (Fig. 2).[23] In some patients who have failed previous attempts at midface lifting, or when topography or skin shortage is pervasive, skin grafting still has role in surgical correction (Fig. 3). Scarring after such surgery may be mitigated by injections of the antimetabolite 5-fluorouracil (5FU).[24] Harvesting of skin from the supraclavicular area with appropriate thinning of subcutaneous tissue has shown to be effective in enhancing donor match and transition to lower lid skin.[1,24] Finally, in patients with true or relative globe prominence

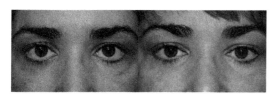

Fig. 1. A 36-year-old woman who presented with bilateral lower eyelid retraction 7 months following transcutaneous lower eyelid blepharoplasty (*left*). Note her improved lower eyelid position 3 months after lower eyelid volume augmentation (*right*). She was very satisfied with the outcome. (*From* Griffin G, Azizzadeh BA, Massry GG. New Insights into Physical Findings Associated with Post Blepharoplasty Lower Eyelid Retraction. *Aesth Surg J* 2014;34:995-1004; with permission.)

and in those with orbicularis deficit, orbital decompression by itself, or as an adjunct to MSC, has shown promise in helping to correct lower lid retraction in Graves' disease patients and also in patients with PBLER (**Fig. 4**).[25,26] The authors refer to this as orbital surgical vector correction. By setting the globe back, the vector discrepancy is reduced and a compromised orbicularis works less to maintain eyelid position. This is very specialized surgery that should only be addressed with a surgeon well-versed in decompression surgery. Because discussion of these alternate interventions can be a separate article within itself, please refer to references for detailed descriptions of each.[1,23–27]

PBLER presents with the characteristic findings of retracted (pulled down) lower lids, scleral show (sclera noted between inferior iris and lower lid margin), and rounded lateral canthi.[1,21] Typical ancillary findings include a shortened horizontal palpebral fissure without animation[1] and fishmouthing (medial displacement of the lateral canthus) with attempted eyelid closure.[1,21]

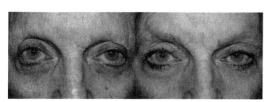

Fig. 2. A woman in her 70s developed bilateral lower eyelid retraction following transcutaneous lower blepharoplasty (*left*). Postoperative photograph 1 year after a minimally invasive orbicularis-sparing (MIOS) lower eyelid recession procedure demonstrating improved lower eyelid position (*right*). (*From* Yoo DB, Griffin GR, Azizzadeh BA, Massry GG. The Minimally Invasive Orbicularis Sparing "MIOS" Lower Eyelid Recession Procedure for Mild to Moderate Lower Lid Retraction with Reduced Orbicularis Strength. *JAMA Facial Plast Surg.2014*;16(2):140-146.)

Fishmouthing is related to poor lateral canthal fixation and leads to a biomechanical limitation of eyelid closure.[1,28,29] To best assess PBLER, a basis of understanding of normal native lower eyelid position is essential. The lower eyelids are anchored by the canthal tendons medially and laterally, and supported from below by eyelid or orbital fat and the bony and soft tissue projection of the midface. Anteriorly, the lower lid is supported by the dynamic sphincteric function of the orbicularis muscle, and by having an adequate amount of vertical eyelid skin to span the cheek to the lower eyelid margin.[12,19–21] When any of these parameters is negatively affected, eyelid retraction can occur. The authors use a standard examination protocol for patients with PBLER. This includes identifying the presence and degree of 6 potential distinct deficits.[21] The following sections list these problems and how their presence is evaluated. Also, the percentage of occurrence of these findings on examination has been studied by the authors,[21] and their experience is elaborated for each.

Orbicularis Strength

To test orbicularis strength, the patient is asked to close their eye forcefully. In the normal setting, the examiner should not be able to pry the lid open. If the examiner can, then orbicularis weakness is present. This can be subjectively graded on a 1+ (minimal) to 4+ (maximal) scale. Orbicularis deficit occurs in 86% of eyelids (**Fig. 5**A, B).[21]

Internal Eyelid Scar

Internal eyelid scar is assessed with the forced traction test (FTT). With the patient looking up, the lower eyelid is pushed superiorly. It should move freely to the upper lid. If there is more than mild restriction of superior lid excursion, the test is positive and can signify an internal eyelid scar (**Fig. 5**C, D). Anterior lamellar shortage can also limit excursion, so the deficit must be out of proportion to skin shortage. This can be differentiated by elevating the cheek and then performing the FTT. The cheek elevation will eliminate the anterior lamellae deficit by recruitment of skin from below. The authors refer to this maneuver as the FFT2 (**Fig. 6**). An internal eyelid scar of clinical significance occurs in 17% of eyelids.[21] Of note, the authors use the term internal eyelid scar as opposed to the traditional middle lamellar scar because the middle lamella refers to the orbital septum. It has been recently shown that orbital septal violation, in and of itself, does not lead to eyelid scars of clinical significance.[30] Instead, a mixed skin, muscle, and septal scars are most likely the culprits.

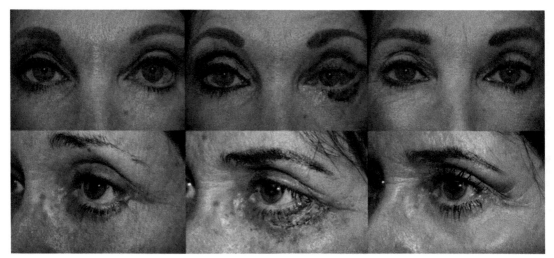

Fig. 3. Two women in their 60s underwent skin grafting procedures to their left lower eyelids for lower eyelid retraction after transcutaneous blepharoplasty; preoperative (*left top* and *bottom*). The first patient's (*top row*) donor site was the same-side upper eyelid. The second patient's (*bottom row*) donor site was the supraclavicular area. Just before removing skin graft sutures at 1 week (*top middle*). Two weeks postoperative, with sutures removed (*bottom middle*). The final postoperative outcome at 9 months (*right top* and *bottom*). (*From* Yoo DB, Azizzadeh BA, Massry GG. Injectable 5FU With or Without Added Steroid in Periorbital Skin Grafting: Initial Observations. *Opthal Plast Reconst Surg.* 2015;31:122-26; with permission.)

Anterior Lamellar (Skin or Muscle) Shortage

Anterior lamellar shortage is tested by having the patient look up and open their mouth. If increased retraction or frank ectropion develops, tissue shortage exists. This can also be graded on a similar 1 + to 4 + subjective scale by the examiner. Anterior lamella shortage was found in 79% of eyelids (**Fig. 7**A, B).[21]

Volume Loss to Inferior Orbit or Eyelid

Volume loss to the inferior orbit or the eyelid is evaluated subjectively by observing significant hollowing (concavity) of the inferior eyelid. This occurs in 70% of eyelids (**Fig. 7**C, D).[21]

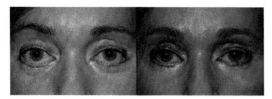

Fig. 4. A 57-year-old woman developed severe post-blepharoplasty lower eyelid retraction after transcutaneous blepharoplasty. She underwent several lower eyelid and canthal revisional procedures without improvement (*left*). After bilateral orbital decompression combined with standard MSC surgery, she attained an excellent result 10 months postoperative (*right*).

Negative Vector Topography of Globe to Cheek (Negative Vector Eyelid)

The patient is evaluated in sagittal view. If the tip of the cornea project more anteriorly than the midface, a negative vector eyelid is present. This occurs in 65% of eyelids (**Fig. 7**E, F).[21]

Eyelid Laxity

Eyelid laxity is evaluated by eyelid snap and distraction testing. In the snap test, the lower lid is pulled inferiorly by the examiner and then released (**Fig. 8**A). The eyelid should return to its native position quickly and without blink. If this does not occur the test is abnormal (positive snap). In the distraction test, the lower lid is pulled away from the globe (**Fig. 8**B). If the eyelid can be pulled 8 mm or more from the cornea, then the test is abnormal (positive). Both tests evaluate eyelid laxity, with the snap test more a measure of orbicularis tone and the distraction test more a measure of canthal tendon integrity. Eyelid laxity occurs in 62% of eyelids.[21]

It is important to know that PBLER is rarely caused by 1 deficit in isolation. In the authors' study, most patients had 4 to 5 obvious deficits, and there was a direct correlation of number of deficits and amount of eyelid retraction.[21] Therefore, even with its limitation noted (patient satisfaction), most of the authors' patients still undergo standard MSC surgery (because it addresses 3

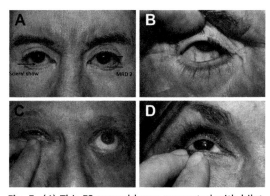

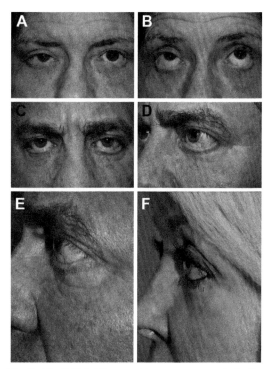

Fig. 5. (*A*) This 52-year-old man presented with bilateral lower eyelid retraction following lower eyelid transcutaneous blepharoplasty. Note the bilateral inferior scleral show. The marginal reflex distance (MRD)2 is the measured distance (mm) between the cornea light reflex and the central lower eyelid margin. (*B*) The eyelid is opened by the examiner on attempted forceful closure of the eyelid by the patient, demonstrating significant orbicularis weakness. (*C*) A 64-year-old man presented with lower eyelid retraction after transcutaneous lower blepharoplasty with minimally limited forced eyelid elevation. Internal eyelid scarring (which will limit forced eyelid elevation) is assessed by the forced eyelid traction test (FTT) in which the lower eyelid is displaced superiorly by the examiner. (*D*) A 68-year-old woman presented with lower eyelid retraction 9 months following transcutaneous lower blepharoplasty. Note moderate amount of reduced forced eyelid elevation. (*From* Griffin G, Azizzadeh BA, Massry GG. New Insights into Physical Findings Associated with Post Blepharoplasty Lower Eyelid Retraction. *Aesth Surg J* 2014;34:995-1004; with permission.)

critical issues). Before surgery, however, all patients are counseled about the expected outcome and how this outcome is perceived by patients in terms of satisfaction. Mitigating expectations realistically has increased postoperative success

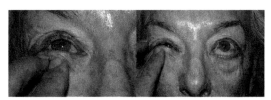

Fig. 6. A woman in her 70s has a FTT (*left*), which is limited (positive). Besides an internal eyelid scar, this can be related to anterior lamellar deficit. This can be identified when the cheek is lifted to recruit skin from below and then forcibly lifting the eyelid (*right*). The authors refer to this as the FFT2. If the FTT is positive (limited eyelid elevation) and the FTT2 is negative (lower eyelid displaces superiorly) then the deficit is primarily anterior lamellar. In many cases there is a mixed picture.

Fig. 7. (*A, B*) This 57-year-old woman presented after transcutaneous lower blepharoplasty. A skin deficit was evident in **Fig. 7**B when she looked upward with her mouth ajar (note lower eyelids pull down further). (*C, D*) This 56-year-old man with lower eyelid retraction after transcutaneous lower blepharoplasty demonstrates inferior eyelid/orbit volume deficit. (*E*) The same patient in 7D showing negative vector eyelid configuration. (*F*) A 62-year-old woman with a similar history as patient 7 C, D, E also has a negative-vector eyelid configuration. (*From* Griffin G, Azizzadeh BA, Massry GG. New Insights into Physical Findings Associated with Post Blepharoplasty Lower Eyelid Retraction. *Aesth Surg J* 2014;34:995-1004; with permission.)

greatly.[1] When the primary dominant examination findings are volume loss, vector discrepancy, and/or orbicularis deficit, the alternate interventions previously noted are suggested as first-line treatment. Also, although posterior spacer grafts have been a mainstay of standard MSC surgery, the authors have used them less frequently over the last 5 years. Only 17% of patients in the authors' previous evaluation of PBLER patients had an internal eyelid scar of clinical significance,[21] which was much less than anticipated. In the past, this has been a primary indication for using eyelid spacers. However, the authors think spacer grafts likely also improve eyelid contour, potentially add eyelid volume, and are useful in posterior lamellar lengthening in cases of prominent eyes.[31,32] For these reasons, the authors still use

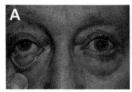 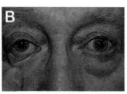

Fig. 8. (*A*) The snap-back test: the lower eyelid is pulled inferiorly and away from the globe. If the eyelid does not snap back to its normal position without blink, the test is positive and eyelid laxity is present. (*B*) The eyelid distraction test: the lower eyelid is pulled away from the globe. If the distance created between the eyelid and globe is 8 mm or more, this signifies eyelid laxity. (*From* Kossler A, Massry G. The Spectrum of Canthal Suspension Techniques in Lower Blepharoplasty. In: Azizadeh B, Murphy M, Johnson C, Massry G, Fitzgerald. *Master Techniques in Facial Rejuvenation.* Elsevier, New York, NY, 2018:152-165.)

spacer grafts frequently. Finally, in the setting of PBLER, before any intervention ocular health is considered, special attention given to vision, the integrity of the cornea, and control of exposure symptoms. It is best to refer to an ophthalmologist to manage symptoms, optimize eye health, and clear the eyes for surgery.

SURGERY (STANDARD MIDFACE LIFTING, SPACER GRAFTS, AND CANTHAL SUSPENSION)

Most surgeries are performed under general anesthesia, especially if a palate graft is harvested. The procedure described is for 1 eyelid; however, surgery is performed bilaterally as dictated by the physical findings on examination. Often, in bilateral cases, we add a temporal brow lift (our preference is an endoscopic approach). In our experience, this alleviates the canthal bunching that can occur in the first 2 to 3 months postoperatively. It also aesthetically smooths the transition between the cheek, lateral eyelid, and temple. In this setting, the temporal brow is addressed (as has been discussed preciously).[33,34] The CS is typically performed in an open fashion, which is described. Less frequently, a closed CS is performed. Please refer to references of this procedure for description.[35–37]

The canthus, lower eyelid, and midface are anesthetized with 3 mL of 1% xylocaine with 1:100:000 epinephrine. Next, a canthotomy and cantholysis are performed. A subtarsal incision is made the full width of the lower eyelid through both the conjunctiva and lower eyelid retractors. These tissues are engaged with a 4-0 silk traction suture, which is secured to the head drape. A

Desmarres retractor is placed to displace the lower lid inferiorly. Blunt cotton-tip dissection ensues in the postorbicularis fascial plane to the orbital rim. In these reoperations, this is often a scarred plane. The Desmarres retractor can be used to sweep the surgical plane inferiorly to aid in dissection. If blunt dissection is not possible (eg, in the setting of severe scar), the Desmarres retractor is elevated, which pulls the lower eyelid up, placing the surgical plane on stretch, and an electrocautery unit or a Stevens scissors is used to dissect between the orbicularis muscle and a true or pseudo orbital septum to the orbital rim. The orbital rim should be isolated from the medial to the lateral canthus. The arcus marginalis is identified and midface dissection ensues. There are 2 surgical planes for midface surgery: subperiosteal or preperiosteal. Our preference is preperiosteal for a few reasons. First, this creates a plane where there are raw surfaces above and below, which can lead to a better adhesion and permanency of the lift. Also, if the cheek soft tissue is mobile over underlying bone (ie, positive glide), when the periosteum is elevated and refixated superiorly, the soft tissue of the cheek may still glide inferiorly, as was the case preoperatively. The midface dissection begins laterally as the orbitomalar ligament is released just above the periosteum in the deep suborbicularis oculi fat (SOOF) plane. It is important to stay in a deep plane to leave as much soft tissue above as possible. This reduces the incidence of skin pucker when engaging the midface for lifting. Dissection ensues laterally to the canthus and medially typically to the junction of the SOOF and medial lip elevators (levator labii superioris and alaeque nasi). We have rarely needed to release these muscles for added lift. Once the orbitomalar ligament is cut, blunt dissection with a cotton-tip proceeds to the zygomatic ligament. Depending on the degree of cheek mobilization and lift needed, this ligament can also be incised. Finger dissection in a sweeping fashion bluntly releases any soft tissue bands that may limit the cheek lift. A 4-0 prolene suture is used to engage the SOOF of the midface. This is a critical step in surgery and some nuances apply. A sweet spot for tissue engagement is critical. The authors prefer the inferior nasal SOOF because we think this best redirects the vector of the midface superolaterally, which is the most anatomic lift. Three close-proximity suture bites of the SOOF are usually taken for security of midface engagement. Finally, the prolene suture is secured to either the lateral orbital rim periosteum or the deep temporalis fascia (DTF) above (dictated by surgeon preference and tissue integrity), to secure the midface. The terminal preseptal orbicularis is

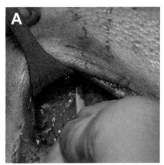 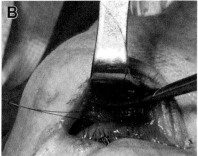 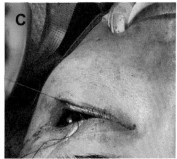

Fig. 9. (*A*) Transconjunctival approach to midface lifting. The cotton-tip is pointing to the preperiosteal midface dissection plane. Note orbital fat above, just below surgical glove. (*B*) The SOOF of the midface is engaged with 4-0 prolene suture. (*C*) Suture elevating the midface in a superolateral vector to recruit skin for the lower eyelid.

then engaged with a 4-0 Vicryl suture on a half-circled P-2 needle and secured to the periosteum or the DTF to create a biplanar (deep SOOF and more superficial orbicularis) suspension of the midface. The Vicryl (polyglactin 910) suture (Ethicon US LLC, Cincinnati, OH) is used because it dissolves and had less tendency to be felt or seen through then skin just lateral to the canthus.

Attention is now brought to the hard palate. An adult-sized Jennings mouth retractor is placed to open the mouth. The hard palate is injected with 1 to 2 cubic centimeters (ccs) of the same local anesthetic. The key with injection is to note whitening (blanching) of the normally red mucosa. The graft size is demarcated based on the degree of retraction and the lower eyelid contour deficit identified preoperatively. When marking the hard palate for harvest, the authors prefer to stay a few millimeters lateral to the medial raphe and medial to the root of the teeth. Further, the dissection should start as close to the central incisors as possible. This allows a longer graft (as much as 30 mm) when needed. The graft can be harvested with a scalpel blade or other cutting device per surgeon preference. Dissection is in the fibrofatty submucosal plane. Hemostasis is attained with cautery, application of Monsel solution, and Surgicel Original Hemostat (Ethicon, Arlington, TX, USA). A prefabricated dental retainer is placed at the conclusion of the graft harvest. The graft is then cut to size and thinned appropriately. The graft is sewn to the tarsus above and the conjunctiva and retractors below with interrupted and buried 6-0 plain gut suture. Before placing the graft, the retractors can be recessed off the conjunctiva (true retractor recession).[23] We add this step in more severe cases of retraction, especially when the cicatricial component is greater or the globe midface vector discrepancy is more significant. For surgeons first performing this surgery, the palate graft can be placed before midface suspension because surgical exposure may be better. The terminal canthus is then secured to the inner orbital rim periosteum with a 4-0 Vicryl suture on a P-3 needle. Many of these cases have premorbid shortened horizontal palpebral fissures, so lid shortening is rarely needed and mostly avoided. A Frost suture or variant is placed to put the lower eyelid on stretch during the first 1 to 2 weeks of recovery. The authors use a 4-0 silk suture looped over a cotton bolster. The suture passes through the gray line of the lower eyelid and is secured

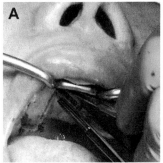 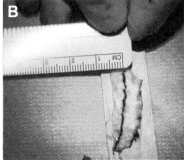 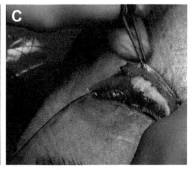

Fig. 10. (*A*) Intraoperative exposure and demarcation of hard palate graft for harvest. (*B*) Customized measured division of palate graft in preparation for implantation. (*C*) Plate graft placed as posterior eyelid space.

through the eyebrows or, alternatively, when a brow lift is added, taped to the forehead with steri-strips over Mastisol Liquie Adhesive (Ferndale IP, Inc, Ferndale, MI, USA). **Figs. 9–11** demonstrate salient features of PBLER surgery, and **Figs. 12–14** show representative examples of results of standard MSC surgery.

POSTOPERATIVE CARE

Patients are instructed to apply ice to the eyelids 10 minutes per hour while awake for 2 days. An antibiotic ointment is applied to sutures and an antibiotic or steroid drop is applied to the eyes 3 times a day for 1 week. The dental retainer is used for comfort as needed and a low sodium soft diet is advanced as tolerated. A topical liquid viscous lidocaine solution is used to gargle with as needed daily for comfort. This can be alternated with an over-the-counter antiseptic solution. Oral antibiotics are used for 1 week, and patients are asked to sleep with the head of the bed at 30° or elevated on 2 pillows for 1 week. The Frost and remaining sutures are removed at 1 to 2 weeks after surgery.

COMPLICATIONS

Prolonged bruising and swelling are not uncommon and require reassurance and, less commonly, oral steroids. Reduced field of vision, inability to read, suture skin erosions, corneal abrasions, and claustrophobia can all occur related to the Frost suture. Early suture removal is indicated if symptoms are more than mild. Eyelid infection is rare but can occur, especially in more compromised eyelids (more previous surgeries with subsequent scaring and poor vascularity). They are treated as clinically indicated with oral antibiotics.

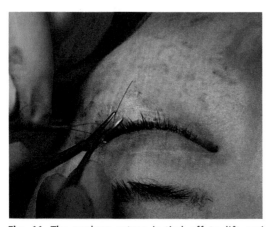

Fig. 11. The prolene suture is tied off to lift and secure the midface.

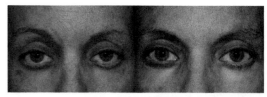

Fig. 12. A 35-year-old woman developed lower eyelid retraction after transcutaneous lower eyelid blepharoplasty (*left*). Note her improvement 2 years after bilateral transeyelid midface lift, implantation of a hard palate graft, and open CS (*right*). In addition, a conservative posterior approach ptosis repair was added.

A cat-eyed appearance is normal and typically resolves within 3 months. Rarely, in relatively enophthalmic patients, the cat-eyed appearance can persist indefinitely. This can be hard to reverse. Fortunately, patients with enophthalmic globe configuration are less prone to retraction. Chemosis is not uncommon because lymphatic drainage is through the canthus (often already disorganized and violated from previous surgeries). In addition, inferior fornix manipulation can further predispose to chemosis (stay high, just below the tarsus, when placing palate graft). Treatment can include lubrication, patching, additional tarsorrhaphy, topical and/or oral steroids, and conjunctival cutdown or cautery. Most cases resolve with conservative measures. Discrepancies in canthal or lower lid height are not uncommon early, and most cases resolve over time. Reoperation to adjust the canthus or trim the palate graft should wait a minimum of 6 months.

On rare occasions, postoperative bleed at the palate donor site can occur. Office cautery with Surgicel (Ethicon US LLC, Cincinnati, OH) packing and pressure application with the retainer usually resolves the issue. If not, cautery in the operating room is required. Donor site infection is rare on antibiotics. If present and persistent, referral or consultation with a dentist is

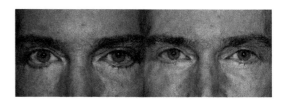

Fig. 13. A 59-year-old man had previous transcutaneous lower blepharoplasty with subsequent lower eyelid retraction, and then numerous revisional lower eyelid can canthal procedures that did not meet his expectations (*left*). One-year status after standard MSC surgery (*right*). Note improved lower eyelid position, canthal angle appearance.

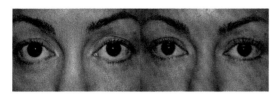

Fig. 14. A 34-year-old woman developed lower lid retraction after transcutaneous lower blepharoplasty. She presented with the classic findings of lower eyelid retraction, inferior scleral show, and rounded canthi (*left*). One year after standard MSC surgery (closed CS), all deficits improved significantly (*right*).

warranted. Similar referral is needed when rare granulation tissue irregularities occur on the hard palate donor site. On occasion, neuropathic pain on the roof of the mouth can occur. This is cumbersome and can resolve with tricyclic antidepressants (Elavil), gabapentinoids (Lyrica, Neurontin), or time.

Late regression of effect is unfortunate and most likely related to undercorrection (incidence goes down with experience) or tissue biology (wound contraction). Injections of wound modulators such as 5FU or steroid preparations and tissue expansion with hyaluronic acid gels are useful if timely.[38] Finally, canthal irregularities (eg, webs, commissure separation, scars) can occur with any surgeon but occur especially in less experienced hands. These are very difficult to correct.[39,40] The authors have found that strict attention to surgical technique, reduction of tissue trauma, recreation of anatomy, and experience are the best methods of prevention.

SUMMARY

PBLER is a devastating complication primarily seen after transcutaneous lower eyelid surgery. Because the surgical dictum is do no harm, and this complication occurs after an elective cosmetic procedure that alters both form and function, patients often feel harmed. This emotional overlay adds a psychological component to an already difficult problem to address. Add this to the unpredictability of this complex revision surgery and it becomes clear that meeting patient expectations is difficult at best. For these reasons, these cases should not be taken lightly and referral to a surgeon who has experience with them is important. Even in this scenario, patients should be educated well regarding expectations. Fortunately, advances in more contemporary surgical and nonsurgical modalities continue to emerge that may lead to higher patient satisfaction. Keeping abreast of these changes and the ongoing developing

literature regarding PBLER is essential for surgeons who choose to take on these cases.

On a final note, as surgeons, we have focused on an improvement in eyelid position as the primary endpoint of PBLER surgery. What the authors have found is that elevating the lower eyelid, although of primary importance, is just 1 component of PBLER repair that patients focus on. The authors think it is also very important to pay attention to the appearance of the canthal angle and the length of the horizontal palpebral aperture when planning surgery on these patients. Addressing these additional deficits, or at least providing preoperative counseling regarding limitations in outcome related to them, has significantly improved the authors' success rate with surgery.

REFERENCES

1. Massry GG. Contemporary Thoughts On Post-Blepharoplasty Lower Lid Retraction. 3rd Triennial Multidisciplinary Masters' Symposium On Blepharoplasty And Facial Rejuvenation. Sydney, Australia, September 2, 2017.
2. Ferri M, Oestreicher JH. Treatment of post-blepharoplasty lower eyelid retraction by free tarsoconjunctival grafting. Orbit 2002;21:281–8.
3. Rosenberg DB, Lattman J, Shah AR. Prevention of lower eyelid malposition after blepharoplasty: anatomic and technical considerations of the inside-out blepharoplasty. Arch Facial Plast Surg 2007;9(6):434–8.
4. Marshak H, Morrow DM, Dresner SC. Small incision preperiosteal midface lift for correction of lower eyelid retraction. Ophthalmic Plast Reconstr Surg 2010;26:176–81.
5. Edgerton MT Jr. Causes and prevention of lower lid ectropion following blepharoplasty. Plast Reconstr Surg 1972;49:367–73.
6. Webster RC, Davidson TM, Reardon EJ, et al. Suspending sutures in blepharoplasty. Arch Otolaryngol 1979;105:601–4.
7. Patipa M. The evaluation and management of lower eyelid retraction following cosmetic surgery. Plast Reconstr Surg 2000;106:438–53.
8. Carraway JH, Mellow CG. The prevention and treatment of lower lid ectropion following blepharoplasty. Plast Reconstr Surg 1990;85(6):971.
9. Shorr N, Goldberg RA, Eshaghian B, et al. Lateral canthoplasty. Ophthal Plast Reconstr Surg 2003; 19(5):345.
10. Fagien S. Algorithm for canthoplasty: the lateral retinacular suspension: a simplified suture canthopexy. Plast Reconstr Surg 1999;103(7):2042–58.
11. Chong KK, Goldberg RA. Lateral canthal surgery. Facial Plast Surg 2010;2693:193–200.

12. Massry GG. Comprehensive lower eyelid rejuvenation. Facial Plast Surg 2010;26(3):209–21.
13. Shorr N, Fallor MK. "Madame butterfly" procedure: combined cheek and lateral canthal suspension procedure for post-blepharoplasty, "round eye," and lower eyelid retraction. Ophthal Plast Reconstr Surg 1985;1(4):229.
14. Patel BCK, Patipa M, Anderson RL, et al. Management of postblepharoplasty lower eyelid retraction with hard palate spacer grafts and lateral tarsal strip. Plast Reconstr Surg 1997;99:1251–60.
15. Korn BS, Kikkawa DO, Cohen SR, et al. Treatment of lower eyelid malposition with dermis fat grafting. Ophthalmology 2008;115:744–51.e2.
16. Taban M, Douglas R, Li T, et al. Efficacy of "thick" acellular human dermis (alloderm) for lower eyelid retraction. Arch Facial Plast Surg 2005;7:38–44.
17. Shorr N. Madame Butterfly procedure with hard palate graft: management of postblepharoplasty round eye and scleral show. Facial Plast Surg 1994;10:90–118.
18. Anderson RL, Gordy DD. The tarsal strip procedure. Arch Ophthalmol 1979;97:2192–6.
19. Massry GG. Managing the lateral canthus in the aesthetic patient. In: Massry GG, Murphy M, Azizzadeh BA, editors. Master techniques in blepharoplasty and periorbital rejuvenation. New York: NY Springer; 2011. p. 185–97.
20. Kossler A, Massry G. The spectrum of canthal suspension techniques in lower blepharoplasty. In: Azizadeh B, Murphy M, Johnson C, et al, editors. Master techniques in facial rejuvenation. New York: Elsevier; 2018. p. 152–65.
21. Griffin G, Azizzadeh BA, Massry GG. New insights into physical findings associated with post blepharoplasty lower eyelid retraction. Aesthet Surg J 2014;34:995–1004.
22. Massry GG. A comparison of patient and surgeon satisfaction in revisional aesthetic eyelid and periorbital surgery. Presented at the 44th annual fall meeting of the American Society of Ophthalmic Plastic and Reconstructive Surgery. New Orleans, LA, November 8, 2013.
23. Yoo DB, Griffin GR, Azizzadeh BA, et al. The minimally invasive orbicularis sparing "MIOS" lower eyelid recession procedure for mild to moderate lower lid retraction with reduced orbicularis strength. JAMA Facial Plast Surg 2014;16(2):140–6.
24. Yoo DB, Azizzadeh BA, Massry GG. Injectable 5FU with or without added steroid in periorbital skin grafting: initial observations. Ophthalmic Plast Reconstr Surg 2015;31:122–6.
25. Pieroni Goncalves AC, Gupta S, Monteiro MLR, et al. Customized minimally invasive orbital decompression surgery improves lower eyelid retraction and contour in thyroid eye disease. Ophthalmic Plast Reconstr Surg 2017;33(6):446–51.
26. Taban RM. Expanding role of orbital decompression in aesehtic surgery. Aesthet Surg J 2017;37:3889–95.
27. Massry GG. Lower eyelid retraction: my approach and thinking. Advanced aesthetic blepharoplasty, midface and contouring 2017. St Petersburg (Russia).
28. McCord CD, Miotto GC. Dynamic diagnosis of "fishmouthing" syndrome, an overlooked complication of blepharoplasty. Aesthet Surg J 2013;33:497–504.
29. McCord CD, Walrath JD, Nahai F. Concepts in eyelid biomechanics with clinical implications. Aesthet Surg J 2013;33:209–21.
30. Schwarcz R, Fezza J, Jacono A, et al. Stop blaming the septum. Ophthal Plast Reconstr Surg 2016;32:49–52.
31. Taban M. Lower eyelid retraction surgery without internal spacer graft. Aesthet Surg J 2017;37:133–6.
32. Massry GG. Commentary on: lower eyelid retraction surgery without internal spacer graft. Aesthet Surg J 2017;33:137–9.
33. Massry GG. The Temporal Endo-Style Brow Lift: Why This Is My Preference. Facial Surgery 2 Session. The Annual Vegas Cosmetic Surgery Meeting. An International Multispecialty Symposium. Las Vegas, Nevada, June 8, 2018.
34. Stalworth CL, Wang TD. Endoscopic brow and forehead rejuvenation. In: Massry GG, Murphy M, Azizzadeh B, editors. Master techniques in blepharoplasty and periorbital rejuvenation. New York: Springer; 2011. p. 69–78.
35. Massry GG. An argument for closed canthoplasty in aesthetic lower blepharoplasty. Ophthalmic Plast Reconstr Surg 2012;28:474–5.
36. Taban M, Nakra T, Hwang C, et al. Aesthetic lateral canthoplasty. Ophthal Plast Reconstr Surg 2010;26:190–4.
37. Georgescu D, Anderson RL, McCann JD. Lateral canthal resuspension sine canthotomy. Ophthal Plast Reconstr Surg 2011;27:371–5.
38. Taban M, Lee S, Hoenig JA, et al. Postoperative wound modulation in aesthetic and eyelid periorbital surgery. In: Massry GG, Murphy M, Azizzadeh BA, editors. Master techniques in blepharoplasty and periorbital rejuvenation. New York: NY Springer; 2011. p. 307–12.
39. Massry GG. Lateral canthal webs. Pearls and pitfalls in cosmetic oculoplastic surgery. New York: Springer New York; 2015. p. 253–5.
40. Massry GG. Cicatricial canthal webs. Ophthal Plast Reconstr Surg 2011;27(6):426–30.

Complications Associated with Fat Grafting to the Lower Eyelid

Robi N. Maamari, MD[a],*, Guy G. Massry, MD[b], John Bryan Holds, MD, FACS[c]

KEYWORDS

- Blepharoplasty complication • Eyelid volume • Fat graft • Fat transfer • Fat transplantation
- Lipofilling • Lipogranuloma

KEY POINTS

- Techniques of facial fat transfer or fat grafting can produce serious periorbital complications.
- Complications of lower eyelid fat grafting are largely technique related, allowing avoidance by appropriate surgical technique.
- Characteristic patterns of fat grafting complications above and below the orbital rim demand specific approaches to treatment.
- Effective techniques are available for the treatment of complications of lower eyelid fat grafting.

INTRODUCTION

Autologous fat grafting has gained increased acceptance and utility in the periorbital area for the rejuvenation of the aging face since its description by Coleman in 1995.[1] The technique provides a means of augmenting facial volume, which represents a fundamental shift from the surgical paradigm of the past century, which focused on tissue subtraction via excision of variable amounts of skin, muscle, and fat.[2] Fat grafting, along with fat preservation blepharoplasty (native fat transposition), have led to natural surgical outcomes that avoid the volume-deficient stigmata of traditional lower blepharoplasty, and focus on the recreation of the curves and contours of youth.[2,3] Fat grafting is used as an adjunct to lower blepharoplasty, or as a stand-alone intervention.[2,4–7] In the periorbita, the primary goal of treatment is effacement of the eyelid/cheek interface with special attention to the tear trough deformity.[8–10] This is accomplished by direct or tissue adjacent fat grafting of these periorbital depressions.[6]

Many complications may occur with fat grafting of the lower eyelid including volume undercorrection or overcorrection, contour irregularities, prolonged bruising and swelling, infection, granulomas and inflammation, and vascular embolization with visual loss or cerebral infarct.[2,11–22] This attention to volumizing the lower eyelid tear trough area creates a subset of patients with overvolumized tear troughs and associated facial deformities who suffer short- and long-term complications. The treatment of these chronically overvolumized patients prompts specific surgical approaches to evaluation and therapeutic procedure.[2,19]

Attention to appropriate principles in patient evaluation and treatment, including safe surgical technique, will avoid most complications of fat grafting in the lower eyelid and periorbital area.

Disclosure: Drs G.G. Massry and J.B. Holds received royalties from Elsevier, Springer. Dr G.G. Massry received royalties from Quality Medical Publishers. Dr R.N. Maamari has nothing to disclose.
[a] John F. Hardesty, MD Department of Ophthalmology and Visual Sciences, Washington University School of Medicine, 660 S. Euclid Avenue, Campus Box 8096, St. Louis, MO 63110, USA; [b] Ophthalmic Plastic and Reconstructive Surgery, 150 N. Robertson Boulevard, Suite 314, Beverly Hills, CA 90211, USA; [c] Ophthalmic Plastic and Cosmetic Surgery, Inc.,12990 Manchester Road, Suite 102, Des Peres, MO 63131-1860, USA
* Corresponding author.
E-mail address: maamarir@wustl.edu

Facial Plast Surg Clin N Am 27 (2019) 435–441
https://doi.org/10.1016/j.fsc.2019.07.001

VOLUMETRIC-RELATED AND CONTOUR-RELATED COMPLICATIONS

Numerous volumetric-related and contour-related abnormalities may be encountered with autologous fat grafting of the lower eyelid, stemming from the diverse surgical techniques across all steps of the procedure. Furthermore, there is no standardized approach to fat preparation, with techniques varying from the injection of minimally or unprocessed suctioned autologous fat to various techniques of drainage, sieving, washing, and centrifuging fat.[14] The short-term and long-term survival of grafted autologous fat is also quite variable, and surgeons must acquire surgical knowledge of the appropriate volumes and surgical technique suited to their own surgical variables and the needs of individual patients.[6,13,23] Failure to appropriately account for these variables results in undercorrection or overcorrection of the lower eyelid tear trough, with inappropriate placement causing other complications.

The Overvolumized Tear Trough

Excessive or inappropriate attention to volumizing the lower eyelid tear trough area creates a subset of patients with overvolumized tear troughs and associated facial deformities that can result in short-term and long-term complications. The treatment of these chronically overvolumized patients prompts specific approaches to evaluation and treatment.

Patient evaluation and prevention

The patients with inappropriately and overvolumized tear troughs and adjacent areas exhibit several characteristic configurations. Common features that the authors have observed from the treatment of these patients is the association of these complications with large injection volumes, surgical technique injecting fat parallel to the tear trough, and the operative use of open-tip Coleman cannulas that are larger and more prone to the injection of larger fat volumes. Intuitively, the injection of fat volumes to the tear trough of greater than 1.5 to 2 mL/side is also more frequently associated with significant overvolumization.

These findings highlight the importance of meticulous surgical technique to limit graft resorption caused by intraoperative traumatic adipocyte damage and postoperative graft necrosis.[23] Precise surgical technique during harvesting, processing, and injecting of the fat graft maximizes the reproducibility and graft survival without requiring aggressive overcorrection, which may result in postoperative complications. During fat harvesting, key technical considerations to increase adipocyte viability include use of manual syringe aspiration with gentle negative pressure instead of conventional high-vacuum liposuction systems and use of larger-diameter harvesting cannulas to limit adipocyte destruction and shear stress, respectively.[24–29] In the fat processing step, it is important to eliminate nonviable free oil droplets, blood, and additional debris to limit their inflammatory effects, which would otherwise increase adipocyte degradation in the graft recipient site.[30] Finally, important considerations during injection into the lower eyelid include use of a small-diameter blunt micro-cannula to minimize trauma to the injection site, strategic tunneling with injection only during withdrawal of the cannula to deposit the fat particles within the preformed tissue plane, and deliberate allocation of only small-diameter fat particles in a fanning pattern to maximize oxygen diffusion across the small diameter fat deposits, minimizing central fat necrosis.[31–35] Typical fat volumes injected near the tear trough are in the 0.02 to 0.04 mL/pass range. Larger volumes per pass are more prone to complication. Attention to these critical surgical techniques reduced the risk of overvolumization of the lower eyelid and the associated complications.

Patient phenotypes seen in overvolumization can be categorized as:

1. Above orbital rim (eyelid)
   a. Discrete large nodule(s): often related to high-volume and bolus injection of fat or focal accumulation of fat owing to intersecting placement tunnels with large local collections of fat.
   b. Multiple small nodules: owing to focal overvolumization, with- or without superficial injection between the skin and orbicularis muscle.
   c. Diffuse: this configuration may result from free dermis fat or pearl fat graft placed retroseptal, or injected fat that is generally localized within the orbicularis muscle or anterior to the orbital septum. Diffuse overvolumization may occur with multiple inappropriate passes, especially paralleling the orbital rim. Injecting parallel to the orbital rim and tear trough is often associated with this complication, and this technique is opposed to the more generally appropriate technique of approaching the inferior orbital rim from below.
2. Below orbital rim
   a. Nodular: more focal fat collections.
   b. Diffuse: entire tear trough and adjacent cheek generally overvolumized. Fat is generally deep to the muscle medially and within the SOOF plane laterally.
3. Combinations of 1 and 2

Surgical Treatment

Patients with chronic complications due to overvolumization in the lower eyelid frequently require surgical treatment of their volume and contour abnormalities. The phenotypic categorization previously noted leads to surgical pearls in treatment.

1. Above orbital rim (eyelid)
   a. Discrete large nodule(s) (**Fig. 1**A): amenable to transconjunctival or transcutaneous (via small stab incision) excision. Generally excised surgically as a distinct nodule of fat that can often be differentiated from the native orbital fat (**Fig. 1**B). The easiest of these overvolumization complications to deal with.
   b. Multiple small nodules (**Fig. 2**A): the least common configuration and the most difficult to treat. May be more amenable to transconjunctival excision (**Fig. 2**B). If superficial fat between skin and orbicularis muscle present, "clean up" via small cutaneous incisions may be required.
   c. Diffuse (**Fig. 3**A): transconjunctival approach with horizontal splitting of the orbicularis muscle to expose grafted fat, which will be apparent and can be prolapsed and teased from the muscle (**Fig. 3**C–E). Only modest orbicularis muscle weakness is generally encountered with appropriate surgical technique. Performed properly, dramatic surgical improvement can be achieved (**Fig. 3**B). With diffuse overvolumization, the surgeon may also excise native fat to retro place the grafted fat.
2. Below orbital rim
   a. Nodular: may be able to reach and tease-out via a transcutaneous or transconjunctival approach (**Fig. 4**).
   b. Diffuse: can generally excise medially and consider repositioning of the native orbital fat (if present) or the use of a dermis fat graft if a secondary defect is encountered. Laterally, fat that cannot be readily excised from the SOOF may require cautery ablation or smoothly contoured excision with culling cautery.
3. Combinations of 1 and 2

The Undercorrected Tear Trough

Patient evaluation and prevention

Undercorrection of the tear trough in lower eyelid fat transfer may be the result of inadequate or inappropriate placement of fat during fat grafting.[2,11,20] Importantly, this risk of postoperative undercorrection and the possible need for

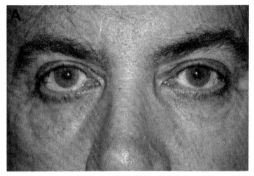
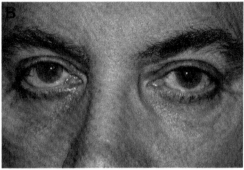

Fig. 1. (*A*) A patient with a discrete large nodule of grafted fat in the right lower lid before transconjunctival revision surgery. (*B*) The same patient after transconjunctival surgical revision.

additional sessions of fat transfer should be thoroughly discussed with the patient during preoperative counseling.

Surgical treatment

Achieving ideal outcomes should always be the targeted goal, but conservative fat grafting of the lower eyelid with small volumes is advised, because this is more easily addressed with surgical revision, relative to the more invasive treatments to correct overvolumization.[20] These approaches to lower eyelid undercorrection include repeat fat grafting, volumization with hyaluronic acid gel fillers, or techniques of surgical fat repositioning using lower eyelid fat.[7,13,14,36]

OTHER COMPLICATIONS

Several additional perioperative and postoperative complications may be encountered with lower eyelid fat transfer, ranging from minor, transient issues to more severe debilitating and disfiguring complications. When performing periocular fat transfer, constant awareness of presenting features and management strategies is necessary to minimize the occurrence of these unwanted complications.

Postoperative ecchymosis prevention begins with preoperative instructions to temporarily

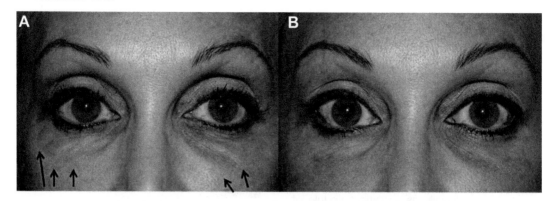

Left = Black Arrows = Lumps/Bumps From Eyelid Fat Grafting
Right = After Surgical Correction "The Most Difficult Eyelid Surgery

Fig. 2. (*A*) A patient with multiple small nodules. The arrows point to multiple lumps and bumps due to inappropriate grafted fat, largely in the orbicularis muscle. (*B*) The same patient after transconjunctival surgical revision with improvement in multiple areas of inappropriate eyelid contour due to grafted fat.

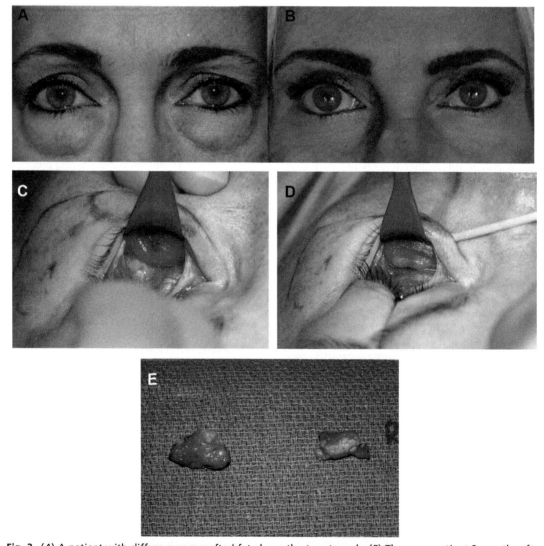

Fig. 3. (*A*) A patient with diffuse excess grafted fat above the tear trough. (*B*) The same patient 3 months after transconjunctival excision of grafted fat. (*C, D*) Transconjunctival approach to excision of grafted fat showing exposure by horizontally splitting the orbicularis muscle. (*E*) With Desmarres retraction and blunt dissection, the grafted fat is generally removed en bloc.

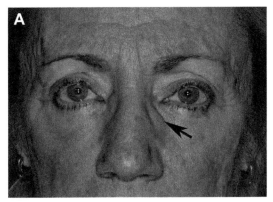 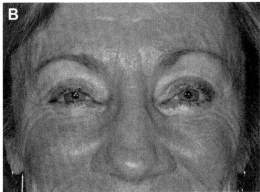

Fig. 4. (*A*) A patient 3 months after 4-lid blepharoplasty and facial fat grafting with a nodule of grafted fat below the orbital rim medially (*arrow*). (*B*) The same patient 1 month after minor room excision under local anesthesia via a 5-mm skin excision over the nodule. A discrete nodule was excised with resolution of the objectional contour anomaly.

discontinue all anticoagulant and antiplatelet therapies, if medically appropriate. In addition, dietary and herbal supplements including vitamin E, fish oil, and *Ginkgo biloba* extracts are stopped before surgery to avoid their increased bleeding risk. Intraoperatively, inadvertent trauma is reduced by ensuring that the harvesting and injection cannulas are withdrawn close to the entry point before pivoting and reinsertion, which limits accidental insertion in the same trajectory.[13,37] Prolonged ecchymosis and edema at the fat grafting sites lasting greater than 2 to 3 weeks are minimized by elevation of the head and application of ice compresses. Periocular bruising at the injection site may be reduced with use of positive pressure systems designed to facilitate capillary collapse to diminish the spread of subcutaneous bleeding. Although placement of ice packs on the injection site can also minimize pain and edema, significant caution must be taken to avoid direct icing because severe cooling may contribute to ischemia and failure of the free fat grafts.[38] Postoperative infections are rarely encountered after autologous fat grafting; however, most surgeons, and the authors, routinely treat patients with prophylactic antibiotics.[19,21]

Undesirable harvest site scars, persistent erythema, and hyperpigmentation can develop at the harvesting cannula entry site.[2] The incidence of these cutaneous findings is reduced with strategic placement of harvest site incisions within the umbilicus or the medial thigh, resulting in discrete surgical sites that are more cosmetically appealing to patients. Furthermore, these entry sites are often subject to high levels of manipulation and distortion to maximize the accessibility of fat graft donor sites, and should be closed with interrupted, nonabsorbable superficial sutures to provide improved dermal wound

apposition to prevent exposure of subcutaneous tissue more prone to granulation. Intralesional injection of triamcinolone (Kenalog) and/or 5-fluorauricil can be used to address persistent granulation or hypertrophic scarring at these entry sites. Sites with nonresolving hyperpigmentation may be treated using topical bleaching creams such as hydroquinone. As a last resort, scar revision may be performed to excise the undesirable scar.

Interestingly, delayed-onset diplopia as a complication of hypertrophy of the fat graft was described in a patient who gained 33 lb over a 2-year period, and ultimately required surgical excision of the hypertrophied fat to improve symptoms.[15] Such hypertrophy of grafted fat is occasionally observed in fat grafts of all sorts, and is a surgical consideration in patients at risk for this.

Serious vision-threatening, and even life-threatening, complications can occur with periorbital fat grafting. Several reports have described irreversible vision loss or stroke after periocular fat grafting caused by retrograde intravascular fat injections through the dorsal, nasal, angular, or supraorbital arteries.[12,18,39] The intravascular fat travels retrograde until the injection is terminated, and then results a fat embolism to the ophthalmic artery, causing permanent blindness, or to the internal carotid artery, causing subsequent embolic cerebral strokes. Preventative techniques include use of a blunt cannula in the periocular area to minimize the risk of inadvertent intra-arterial injections. In addition, small, 1-mL syringes should be used in the periocular area to limit the pressure needed for injection. Finally, fat injection that is only performed as the cannula is being withdrawn reduces the risk of arterial embolism.

SUMMARY

Techniques of facial fat grafting to the lower eyelid and adjacent midface often offer impressive surgical results, but carry risks including early or late undercorrection, prolonged bruising and swelling, infection, granulomas and inflammation, and vascular embolization with visual loss or stroke. Grafted fat may involute with weight loss, or increase to an inappropriate degree should the patient gain weight. Surgical judgment and technique are paramount to achieving excellent results and avoiding complications.

Specific patterns of inappropriate grafted fat are encountered above and below the orbital rim. Recognition of these patterns is helpful to appropriately advise the patient regarding treatment options and to plan surgical revision of these patients. Many cases are amenable to a transconjunctival approach to the inappropriate fat with careful exposure and excision. A limited anterior exposure via a small cutaneous incision may be appropriate in specific cases.

Appropriate and knowledgeable surgical technique to avoid complications is always the best approach. When patients with complications of excess and inappropriate fat grafting are encountered, carefully planned revision surgery can often salvage an acceptable result to the benefit of the patient.

REFERENCES

1. Coleman SR. Long-term survival of fat transplants: controlled demonstrations. Aesthetic Plast Surg 1995;19(5):421–5.
2. Massry G, Azizzadeh B. Periorbital fat grafting. Facial Plast Surg 2013;29(1):46–57. https://doi.org/10.1055/s-0033-1333842.
3. Kossler AL, Peng GL, Yoo DB, et al. Current trends in upper and lower eyelid blepharoplasty among American Society of Ophthalmic Plastic and Reconstructive Surgery members. Ophthalmic Plast Reconstr Surg 2017;1. https://doi.org/10.1097/IOP.0000000000000849.
4. Trepsat F. Periorbital rejuvenation combining fat grafting and blepharoplasties. Aesthetic Plast Surg 2003;27(4):243–53.
5. Serra-Renom JM, Serra-Mestre JM. Periorbital rejuvenation to improve the negative vector with blepharoplasty and fat grafting in the malar area. Ophthalmic Plast Reconstr Surg 2011;27(6):442–6.
6. Stein R, Holds JB, Wulc AE, et al. Phi, fat, and the mathematics of a beautiful midface. Ophthalmic Plast Reconstr Surg 2018;1. https://doi.org/10.1097/IOP.0000000000001167.
7. Einan-Lifshitz A, Holds JB, Wulc AE, et al. Volumetric rejuvenation of the tear trough with repo and ristow. Ophthalmic Plast Reconstr Surg 2013;29(6):481–5.
8. Kim J, Shin H, Lee M, et al. Percutaneous autologous fat injection following 2-layer flap lower blepharoplasty for the correction of tear trough deformity. J Craniofac Surg 2018;1. https://doi.org/10.1097/SCS.0000000000004552.
9. Hamra ST. Arcus marginalis release and orbital fat preservation in midface rejuvenation. Plast Reconstr Surg 1995;96(2):354–62.
10. Kim HS, Choi CW, Kim BR, et al. Effectiveness of transconjunctival fat removal and resected fat grafting for lower eye bag and tear trough deformity. JAMA Facial Plast Surg 2018. https://doi.org/10.1001/jamafacial.2018.1307.
11. Cuzalina A, Guerrero AV. Complications in fat grafting. Atlas Oral Maxillofac Surg Clin North Am 2018;26(1):77–80.
12. Kim J, Kim SK, Kim MK. Segmental ischaemic infarction of the iris after autologous fat injection into the lower eyelid tissue: a case report. BMC Ophthalmol 2017;17(1). https://doi.org/10.1186/s12886-017-0599-8.
13. Kim I, Keller G, Groth M, et al. The downside of fat: avoiding and treating complications. Facial Plast Surg 2016;32(05):556–9.
14. Boureaux E, Chaput B, Bannani S, et al. Eyelid fat grafting: indications, operative technique and complications; a systematic review. J Craniomaxillofac Surg 2016;44(4):374–80.
15. Duhoux A, Chennoufi M, Lantieri L, et al. Complications of fat grafts growth after weight gain: report of a severe diplopia. J Plast Reconstr Aesthet Surg 2013;66(7):987–90.
16. Çetinkaya A, Devoto MH. Periocular fat grafting: indications and techniques. Curr Opin Ophthalmol 2013;24(5):494–9.
17. Park Y-H, Kim KS. Blindness after fat injections. N Engl J Med 2011;365(23):2220.
18. Lee CM, Hong IH, Park SP. Ophthalmic artery obstruction and cerebral infarction following periocular injection of autologous fat. Korean J Ophthalmol 2011;25(5):358.
19. Glasgold RA, Glasgold MJ, Lam SM. Complications following fat transfer. Oral Maxillofac Surg Clin North Am 2009;21(1):53–8.
20. Holck DEE, Lopez MA. Periocular autologous fat transfer. Facial Plast Surg Clin North Am 2008;16(4):417–27.
21. Kranendonk S, Obagi S. Autologous fat transfer for periorbital rejuvenation: indications, technique, and complications. Dermatol Surg 2007;33(5):572–8.
22. Yoon SS, Chang DI, Chung KC. Acute fatal stroke immediately following autologous fat injection into the face. Neurology 2003;61(8):1151–2.

23. Bellini E, Grieco MP, Raposio E. The science behind autologous fat grafting. Ann Med Surg 2017;24: 65–73.

24. Lewis CM. Comparison of the syringe and pump aspiration methods of lipoplasty. Aesthetic Plast Surg 1991;15(1):203–8.

25. Pu LLQ, Coleman SR, Cui X, et al. Autologous fat grafts harvested and refined by the Coleman technique: a comparative study. Plast Reconstr Surg 2008;122(3):932–7.

26. Kirkham JC, Lee JH, Medina MA, et al. The impact of liposuction cannula size on adipocyte viability. Ann Plast Surg 2012;69(4):479–81.

27. Kirkham JC, Lee JH, Austen WG. Fat graft survival: physics matters. Ann Plast Surg 2014;73(3):359.

28. Ozsoy Z, Kul Z, Bilir A. The role of cannula diameter in improved adipocyte viability: a quantitative analysis. Aesthet Surg J 2006;26(3):287–9.

29. Erdim M, Tezel E, Numanoglu A, et al. The effects of the size of liposuction cannula on adipocyte survival and the optimum temperature for fat graft storage: an experimental study. J Plast Reconstr Aesthet Surg 2009;62(9):1210–4.

30. Gutowski KA, ASPS Fat Graft Task Force. Current applications and safety of autologous fat grafts: a report of the ASPS fat graft task force. Plast Reconstr Surg 2009;124(1):272–80.

31. Khouri RK, Rigotti G, Cardoso E, et al. Megavolume autologous fat transfer: part II. Practice and techniques. Plast Reconstr Surg 2014;133(6):1369–77.

32. Khouri RK, Rigotti G, Cardoso E, et al. Megavolume autologous fat transfer: part I. Theory and principles. Plast Reconstr Surg 2014;133(3):550–7.

33. Simonacci F, Bertozzi N, Grieco MP, et al. Procedure, applications, and outcomes of autologous fat grafting. Ann Med Surg 2017;20:49–60.

34. Kakagia D, Pallua N. Autologous fat grafting: in search of the optimal technique. Surg Innov 2014; 21(3):327–36.

35. Coleman SR. Structural fat grafting: more than a permanent filler. Plast Reconstr Surg 2006;118(3 Suppl):108S–20S.

36. Goldberg RA. Transconjunctival orbital fat repositioning: transposition of orbital fat pedicles into a subperiosteal pocket. Plast Reconstr Surg 2000; 105(2):743–8.

37. Butterwick KJ, Nootheti PK, Hsu JW, et al. Autologous fat transfer: an in-depth look at varying concepts and techniques. Facial Plast Surg Clin North Am 2007;15(1):99–111, viii.

38. Bagheri SC, Bohluli B, Consky EK. Current techniques in fat grafting. Atlas Oral Maxillofac Surg Clin North Am 2018;26(1):7–13.

39. Danesh-Meyer HV, Savino PJ, Sergott RC. Ocular and cerebral ischemia following facial injection of autologous fat. Arch Ophthalmol 2001;119:777–8.

Approach to Correction of Septal Perforation

Russell W.H. Kridel, MD[a,b,*], Sean W. Delaney, MD[c]

KEYWORDS

- Rhinoplasty • Septoplasty • Nasal septum • Nasal reconstruction • Iatrogenic

KEY POINTS

- A thorough history, physical examination, and endoscopic measurement of a septal perforation are essential to preoperative assessment and surgical planning for septal perforation repair.
- The relative size of the septal perforation to the surrounding septum is more important than the absolute size of the perforation. Furthermore, as most intranasal mucosal advancement flap methods recruit mucosa from above or below a perforation, a perforation's vertical dimension is more important than its horizontal front-to-back length.
- A surgeon must have a comprehensive understanding of nasal anatomy and physiology, and skill in suturing back in the depths of the nasal cavity to successfully execute these technically challenging septal perforation repairs.

INTRODUCTION

Nasal septal perforations (NSPs), characterized by contiguous defects of the opposing mucoperichondrial flaps and the intervening septal cartilage or bone (**Fig. 1**), present a distinct challenge to the facial plastic surgeon and a nuisance to the patient. The cause of an NSP must be distinguished from a diverse list of potential causes, some of which may be life-threatening[1] (**Table 1**).

Despite the myriad of causes of NSP, previous surgical manipulation of the septum is the most common cause of NSP formation. In a retrospective review of 180 patients undergoing NSP repair, Kridel and Delaney[2] found that previous septorhinoplasty and septoplasty combined accounted for 62.4% of perforations that presented to them. NSPs are commonly formed during or after surgery when corresponding mucosal tears are created, where the intervening septal cartilage or bone has been removed and the septal flaps fail to heal on their own to close the defect. Factors that mitigate septal mucosal blood supply, such as excessive pressure from nasal packing or splinting and septal hematoma formation, can further predispose patients to NSP formation, especially when the septal flaps are already attenuated from chronic rhinitis or prolonged vasoconstrictive nasal spray usage. Perforations may also occur in the postoperative period when a suction tip is inadvertently poked through the septum.[3]

Surgical repair of an NSP can be challenging, requiring the surgeon to operate within the narrow confines of the nasal passages. In addition, the nasal anatomy is often compromised because of previous surgery. The most successful repair techniques involve the tedious and meticulous separation of the components with individual repair of the 3 layers of the septum.[4] As a consequence, NSP repair is an operation that many surgeons completely avoid.[2,5] A thorough understanding of the anatomy and pathophysiology of NSPs, and

Disclosure Statement: The authors have no financial conflicts of interest to disclose.
[a] Facial Plastic Surgery Associates (Private Practice), 6655 Travis Street, Suite 900, Houston, TX 77006, USA;
[b] Division of Facial Plastic Surgery, Department of Otorhinolaryngology - Head and Neck Surgery, McGovern Medical School, University of Texas Health Science Center, Houston, TX, USA; [c] Huntington Ear Nose Throat Head & Neck Specialists (Private Practice), 547 East Union Street, Pasadena, CA 91101, USA
* Corresponding author. Facial Plastic Surgery Associates (Private Practice), 6655 Travis Street, Suite 900, Houston, TX 77006.
E-mail address: rkridel@todaysface.com

Facial Plast Surg Clin N Am 27 (2019) 443–449
https://doi.org/10.1016/j.fsc.2019.07.002
1064-7406/19/© 2019 Elsevier Inc. All rights reserved.

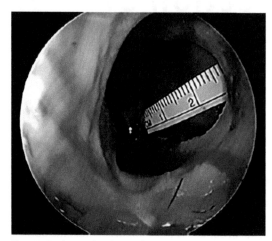

Fig. 1. Endoscopic view of a septal perforation as viewed from the right nasal cavity. A septal perforation comprised a hole in 3 distinct contiguous layers, including both right and left mucoperichondrial flaps and the intervening septal cartilage.

the prognostic factors related to NSP repairs, are crucial to maximization of surgical success. In this article, we review our approach to the correction of the iatrogenic NSP.

CONSIDERATIONS WHEN EVALUATING A SEPTAL PERFORATION

Important factors to consider when approaching the iatrogenic NSP include[1] patient symptoms from the NSP,[2] the size and location of the NSP,[3] the need for revisional rhinoplasty and/or concomitant revision septoplasty maneuvers, and[4] the amount of scarring or loss of other vital anatomic structures that will need to be addressed simultaneously at the time of repair of the NSP.

Perforation Symptoms

Not all patients with NSP require surgical repair. The anticipated benefits of the surgery should be carefully weighed against the potential risks and expense of an attempted repair. Therefore, the decision to undertake an NSP repair depends on whether the patient is symptomatic and whether the surgeon has the skill and experience to perform closure. However, it is a mistake to tell a patient that a small perforation cannot be repaired because the doctor seeing the perforation does not do repairs; a referral to those who routinely do these repairs is, instead, ethically mandated, in case the perforation enlarges years later before the patient finds a physician on his/her own; the perforation could enlarge to the point that it is unrepairable surgically.

Table 1
Causes of nasal septal perforation

Category	Cause
Trauma (iatrogenic)	Nasal surgery, septoplasty, turbinate surgery, rhinoplasty, septal cauterization, septal packing, septal splinting, transsphenoidal surgery, postoperative suctioning, nasotracheal intubation, maxillomandibular advancement surgery
Trauma (external)	Fracture, septal hematoma, piercing injuries
Trauma (self-inflicted)	Nose picking, foreign bodies
Drugs	Vasoconstrictive nasal sprays, steroid nasal sprays, cocaine use, smoking
Chemical irritants	Chromic, sulfuric, and hydrochloric acids, chlorines and bromines, agricultural aerosolized dusts, rice and grain elevator dusts, chemical and industrial dusts, lime, cement, glass, salt, heavy metals, cyanide, arsine
Neoplasm	Adenocarcinoma, squamous cell carcinoma, metastatic carcinoma, midline destructive granuloma
Inflammatory	Vasculitides, collagen vascular diseases, sarcoidosis, granulomatosis with polyangiitis
Infection	Tuberculosis, syphilis, rhinoscleroma, leprosy, rhinosporodiosis, acute fulminant fungal rhinosinusitis, typhoid, diphtheria, septal abscess

Data from Kridel RWH (2004). Considerations in the etiology, treatment, and repair of septal perforations. . *Facial Plast Surg Clin North Am, 12*(04), pp. 435–450.

NSPs vary widely in size, location, and symptomology. Posterior NSPs are generally asymptomatic, small perforations may cause whistling, and anterior, large perforations can result in turbulent airflow that disrupts heat and moisture exchange, reduces olfaction, and desiccates nasal mucosa to create a sensation of obstruction.[2,6–8] For the asymptomatic patient, conservative management with nasal emollients is often all that is necessary. Even mild symptoms, with the exception of nasal obstruction or whistling, can usually be managed nonsurgically. Maintaining nasal moisture can be accomplished with daily application of emollients on cotton-tip applicators. Conversely, those with more symptomatic NSPs may present with complaints of dryness, crusting, epistaxis, rhinorrhea, whistling, pain, or nasal dyspnea. For these patients, surgical interventions may be necessary to improve their quality of life.

Nonsurgical interventions for symptomatic NSPs usually entail nasal emollients and silicone septal buttons. For patients for whom nasal emollients alone are unsuccessful at alleviating their symptoms, who are unwilling to consistently care for their nose, or in whom the sensation of nasal obstruction is dominant, a silicone grommet prosthesis may be considered. Whereas the commercially available prostheses are limited in size and may not fit larger NSPs, custom-made septal buttons are now available and can be made after taking computed tomography measurements. These buttons can sometimes be placed in the office under local anesthesia. This is simplified by the availability of magnetized buttons. For larger perforations, or depending on the tolerance of the patient, sedation may be necessary when placing the prosthesis. While the buttons are in place, regular nasal irrigations are still necessary to maintain the hygiene of the prosthesis. If there is a pre-existing chondritis, the button will not be suitable for treatment of this problem. Septal buttons should also be considered for patients who, for medical reasons, are not good candidates for surgery. In our experience, septal buttons are generally poorly tolerated by patients and are reserved as an alternative for those who do not qualify for, or want, surgery.

The main cause of nasal dyspnea with an NSP is the disruption of lamellar airflow, causing airflow turbulence and the sensation of obstruction.[9] As perforations increase in size, so does the amount of turbulent airflow, thus increasing the incidence of rhinorrhea, which is the nose's attempt to rehydrate itself through secretions. In longstanding perforations, the dried mucosa at their periphery becomes scarred and dysfunctional, losing their cilia and secretory functions. Crust formation and bleeding transpire, progressing to mucosal necrosis and chondritis, which result in enlargement of the NSP, and pain.[2,3] In certain instances, irreversible damage and mucosal atrophy from prolonged turbulent airflow may be so extensive that, despite perforation closure, patients still experience nasal dryness and crusting.[2]

Once the surgeon and patient have decided that the symptoms caused by NSP are significant enough to warrant surgical correction, the surgeon needs to consider the size and location of the septal perforation and the need for concurrent rhinoplasty and/or revision septoplasty.

Perforation Size and Location

When evaluating patients for their surgical candidacy it is essential to measure the perforation, because the size of the NSP is a critical and important prognosticator for closure success. Some patients may present with vast amounts of crusting along the periphery of their NSPs, which are difficult to remove without causing discomfort and bleeding. It may be necessary to have these patients use nasal saline irrigations and emollients for several weeks before surgery to clear the crusts and decrease the inflammation. Once fully visualized, the periphery of the NSP should be palpated with a wet cotton-tip applicator to detect the presence of cartilage close to the perforation edges. Unfortunately, in perforations that occur after septoplasty, there is usually little residual cartilage left, making dissection of the flaps more difficult.

In a systematic review of the literature, Kim and Rhee[10] reported an aggregate closure rate of 93% of NSPs <2 cm and 78% of NSPs >2 cm. A community survey showed a slightly lower success rate of 84%, 64%, and 31% for repairing NSPs <1, 1-2, and >2 cm, respectively.[5] Because most techniques advance surrounding intranasal mucosa to repair NSPs, the difficulty of a repair increases exponentially with the size of an NSP. Small perforations <5 mm can often be closed primarily, whereas larger NSPs require more septal mobilization for a tension-free closure because the septal mucosa has little elasticity.[2,11]

We find that the size of an NSP relative to the surrounding tissue is more important than the absolute size of an NSP. For example, a 1-cm perforation in a child may be much more challenging to repair than a 1.5-cm NSP in an adult with a larger nose and more mucosa available to use for a repair. The vertical dimension is also more important than the anterior-posterior size of a perforation, because most intranasal repair methods recruit tissue from above and below a perforation. Theoretically, an NSP can encompass nearly the length of the septum and still be relatively easy to repair, as long as its vertical dimension is manageable. In Kridel and Delaney's[2] review of 180 patients who underwent NSP repair, 96.7% of those with NSP less than 1.5 cm in height were successfully closed compared with 71.4% of patients with perforations greater than 1.5 cm in the vertical dimension.

Our ability to close large NSPs with local mucosal flaps has been augmented with the use of connective tissue interposition grafts placed between the flaps, which serve as a scaffold for further mucosal ingrowth to close a perforation, even when the mucosal edges cannot be fully apposed.[4] However, there remains a finite limit to the size of an NSP that can be closed using local tissue advancement alone. In the case of the near-total or total NSP, there simply may not be sufficient intranasal tissue available to reapproximate the septal defect. In such cases, the surgeon and patient must have a serious conversation with regard to possible surgical outcomes; some very large septal defects may require a locoregional pedicled flap or microvascular free flap reconstruction that provides vascularized tissue to close the perforation. Whereas these reconstructive efforts enjoy a high rate of successful closure, they do come with a number of associated morbidities. Furthermore, these flaps do not provide respiratory epithelium, and patients must endure chronic nasal dryness and crusting despite a closed NSP.

The location of an NSP is another crucial consideration. Fortunately, for the more symptomatic anterior perforations, one can usually recruit more mucosa from the nasal floor and deep surface of the nasal pyramid than more posterior in the nasal cavity. Because posterior NSPs tend to be less symptomatic, even partial closures can improve patient symptoms considerably.[2] Alternatively, Beckmann and colleagues[12] have reported success in symptom improvement by enlarging NSPs with a posterior septal resection instead, which we generally do not recommend.

Need for Rhinoplasty

External nasal deformities may occur when the NSP cartilage loss involves the L-strut, resulting in tip ptosis, dorsal saddling, and/or columellar retraction,[13] or when there is a suboptimal outcome from a previous rhinoplasty. If such deformities are present, the surgeon may consider a concomitant rhinoplasty and NSP repair, because both operations often share a similar surgical approach, via the open method, to spare the patient a second anesthetic event. The senior author (RWH Kridel) has shown that both primary and revision septorhinoplasty can be safely combined with NSP repair without compromising the perforation closure.[2] However, in the attempt to combine both challenging operations, the surgeon and patient should come to the understanding that the success of NSP closure should be prioritized over any rhinoplasty modifications, which can be performed secondarily and only without compromising the NSP repair. Sometimes, this may mean that additional surgery would be necessary to complete the desired rhinoplasty changes.[14]

As with revision rhinoplasty, it is generally advisable to wait at least a year after a previous rhinoplasty to allow the nose to heal, unless there is a prominent deformity. Most patients with iatrogenic NSP will have little remaining septal cartilage available for harvest. Subsequently, if reconstructive cartilage grafting may be necessary, then nonnasal sources of cartilage should be considered.

SURGICAL REPAIR OF THE SEPTAL PERFORATION

NSP repair should be performed with the aim of restoring normal nasal physiology by recreating laminar airflow, warming and humidification of inspired air, mucus production, and mucociliary transport.

Because an NSP represents a defect in 3 layers, when possible a 3-layered repair should be attempted. In our hands, bilateral intranasal mucosal advancement reinforced by an interposition connective tissue graft has been a reliable repair method that is well accepted by patients. This technique can be performed endonasally, endoscopically, or via an open approach.[5] Intranasal mucosal advancement flaps replace the NSP with physiologic nasal mucosa and obviate the additional external incisions and morbidities associated with locoregional or microvascular free flaps used to close NSP, representing a salient consideration, particularly for the patient who had surgery for cosmetic reasons and who has developed an iatrogenic NSP, and who would be unlikely to accept additional facial incisions or flap-related deformities.

Kridel and Delaney[2] have previously described, in detail, the four-quadrant intranasal mucosal advancement flaps with an interposition connective tissue graft using an external rhinoplasty approach. In brief, the nose is opened up via transcolumellar and marginal incisions. The septal remnant is approached by dissecting between the medial crura, and the mucosal flaps around the NSP are meticulously separated, with care to not to enlarge the NSP (**Fig. 2**). Inferior mucosal advancement flaps are recruited bilaterally, extending from the septum, traversing the nasal floor, and ending under the inferior turbinates, where they are freed from the lateral nasal wall with a back-to-front cut and further mobilized using back cuts to permit advancement medially and a tensionless closure (**Fig. 3**). In addition, superior mucosal advancement flaps are developed by teasing free the mucosa from the undersurface of the upper lateral cartilages and nasal bones in continuity with the superior septal mucosa, allowing for an inferior advancement toward the

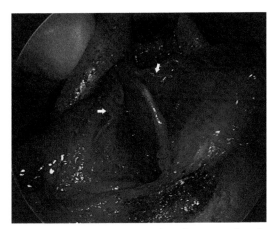

Fig. 2. Using an open approach, submucous detachment of the upper lateral cartilages from the dorsal septum improves exposure and maintains continuity of the septal mucosal flaps that are still attached to the deep surface of the upper lateral cartilages (*arrows*), and recruited for the perforation closure.

perforation (**Fig. 4**). With the extra membrane provided by the flaps, the edges of the perforation on each side are brought together and sewn individually using simple interrupted dissolvable sutures in a posterior-anterior fashion (**Fig. 5**). A connective tissue interposition graft, such as acellular dermis, is placed between the repaired flaps and secured using a continuous quilting stitch to reinforce the repair (**Fig. 6**). Rhinoplasty modifications are next performed only if they can be made without compromising the NSP repair. At the conclusion of the operation, thin Silastic sheets are sutured to the septum on each side to protect the septum

from desiccation and inadvertent trauma from suctioning after the surgery (**Fig. 7**). These sheets are usually removed at about 2 weeks postoperatively after seeing through these transparent sheets that the perforation closure has healed shut.

PREVENTING PERFORATIONS

Benjamin Franklin's axiom *"an ounce of prevention is worth a pound of cure"* holds particular truth with regard to avoiding iatrogenic NSPs. The incidence of iatrogenic septal perforation may be decreased by gentle excision and suture techniques, avoiding or repairing any septal mucosal lacerations at the time of the original surgery, and prophylactically bolstering attenuated mucosal flaps or corresponding mucosal lacerations with interposition grafts.

Because the perichondrium contains much of the vascularity and strength of the mucoperichondrial flaps, it is important that it is included with the elevated flap. Meticulous technique when elevating mucoperichondrial flaps can help preserve the vascularity and viability of septal mucosal flaps. Often because of haste, the novice surgeon will raise mucosal flaps in the improper plane and leave the mucoperichondrium on the septum. Initially, it pays off to spend time making sure that the correct plane is entered; this pays dividends because of less bleeding and decreases the chance of subsequent septal perforation. The vascularity of the mucosal flaps can be further preserved with the use of a quilting stitch to prevent formation of septal hematoma and avoiding overly tight intranasal packing.

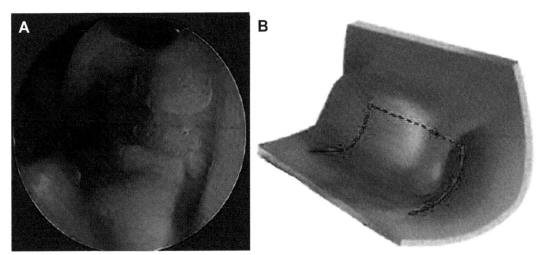

Fig. 3. (*A*) Endoscopic view of the nasal floor mucosal incision, with anterior and posterior back cuts, below the insertion of the left inferior turbinate. (*B*) A schematic representing the mucosal incision used to release the nasal floor mucosal advancement flap laterally.

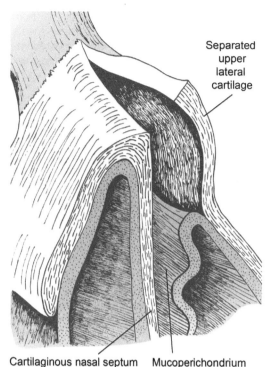

Separated
upper
lateral
cartilage

Cartilaginous nasal septum   Mucoperichondrium
dissected free
from undersurface of ULC

Fig. 4. Taking care to preserve the continuity of the mucosa between the superior septum and the underside of the upper lateral cartilage, a superiorly based bipedicled mucosal flap is developed by carefully teasing free the mucosa on the underside of the upper lateral cartilage to mobilize the flap inferiorly for the perforation closure.

Mucosal lacerations are a common occurrence during septoplasty, especially when one encounters a crooked septum, prominent maxillary crest, or septal spur. The chance of creating inadvertent lacerations are decreased when the mucoperichondrial flaps are first elevated broadly on either side of the septum, crest, or spur. The prominent

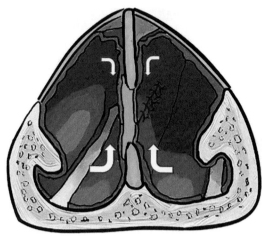

Fig. 6. Illustration demonstrating superiorly and inferiorly based bipedicled mucosal advancement flaps used to close a septal perforation. The nasal floor anterior transverse back-cut is not shown. A connective tissue graft is placed between the septal flaps (green) and sutured to the anterior septum. The septal flaps and interposition grafts are further incorporated using a continuous quilting stitch.

maxillary crest can be a problematic area in which the mucoperiosteum is difficult to elevate. The maxillary crest has a figure-of-T configuration in the coronal plane anteriorly. Attempts to elevate the mucosa off the crest in a superior to inferior fashion often results in a mucosal tear. To avoid this, through the same incision used to approach the caudal septum, a separate mucoperichondrial flap can be elevated along the nasal floor and joined to the septal mucoperichondrial flap to reduce the chance of tearing the adherent mucosa over the crest. In the case of a prominent spur, where the overlying mucosa is already markedly thinned, it is imperative to preserve the continuity of the contralateral mucosal flap. If 1 flap remains

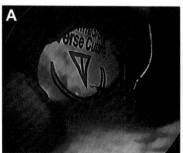
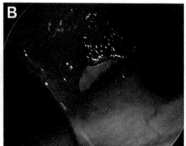
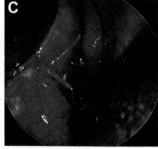

Fig. 5. (*A*) Endoscopic view in the left nasal cavity showing the temporary placement of an intermediary foil between the septal flaps to prevent the needle from inadvertently capturing the contralateral flap. (*B*) The septal flap is closed posterior to anterior using simple interrupted sutures. (*C*) The perforation is closed fully without tension.

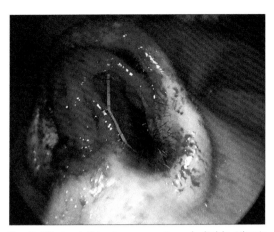

Fig. 7. Bilateral thin, transparent, and pliable Silastic sheets are sutured to the anterior septum to protect the perforation repair and permit direct visualization during the immediate postoperative period. These sheets are usually removed at about 2 weeks postoperatively after observing, through these transparent sheets, that the perforation closure has healed shut.

intact, the chance of creating a perforation is much less.

When attenuated mucosal flaps or corresponding mucosal perforations are encountered, the risk of developing an NSP can be minimized with the placement of morselized cartilage or an interposition connective tissue graft. Even if the crushed cartilage does not survive, it serves as a barrier to prevent NSP formation and may result in fibrosis that strengthens the septum. It may be foolhardy to believe that an NSP created at the time of surgery will heal on its own. It is more likely that the perforation will continue to enlarge, particularly with the cicatricial contraction of healing.[3] If corresponding lacerations are encountered, repair of lacerations at the time of the original surgery can prevent the formation of iatrogenic NSPs and are usually much easier than surgery at a later date.[2]

SUMMARY

Iatrogenic NSP is a dreaded potential, and unfortunately all too common, complication of nasal surgery that causes significant consternation for both surgeon and patient. The decision to operate on an iatrogenic NSP is predicated on the severity of the symptoms related to the perforation, the size, and the location of the NSP. Whereas most NSPs can be successfully repaired using intranasal four-quadrant mucosal advancement flaps with an interposition connective tissue graft, prevention of NSP formation through meticulous

technique, and repair of lacerations at the time of the original surgery is indisputably preferable.

REFERENCES

1. Kridel RWH. Considerations in the etiology, treatment, and repair of septal perforations. Facial Plast Surg Clin North Am 2004;12:435–50.
2. Kridel RWH, Delaney SW. Simultaneous septal perforation repair with septorhinoplasty: a 31-year experience. Facial Plast Surg 2018;34:298–311.
3. Kridel RWH. Considerations in the etiology, treatment, and repair of septal perforations. Facial Plast Surg Clin North Am 2004;12(04):435–50.
4. Kridel RWH, Delaney SW. Discussion: acellular human dermal allograft as a graft for nasal septal perforation reconstruction. Plast Reconstr Surg 2018;141(6):1525–7.
5. Delaney SW, Kridel RWH. Contemporary trends in the surgical management of nasal septal perforations: a community survey. Facial Plast Surg 2018. https://doi.org/10.1055/s-0038-1676049.
6. Kridel RWH. Closure of septal perforation. In: Larrabee WF Jr, Ridgway J, Patel SA, editors. Master techniques in otolaryngology-head and neck surgery: facial plastic surgery. Philadelphia: Wolters Kluwer; 2018. p. 286–95.
7. Cannon DE, Frank DO, Kimbel JS, et al. Modeling nasal physiology changes due to septal perforations. Otolaryngol Head Neck Surg 2013;148(3):513–8.
8. Goh AY, Hussain SS. Different surgical treatments for nasal septal perforation and their outcomes. J Laryngol Otol 2007;121:419–26.
9. Belmont JR. An approach to large nasoseptal perforations and attendant deformity. Arch Otolaryngol Head Neck Surg 1985;111:450–5.
10. Kim SW, Rhee CS. Nasal septal perforation repair: predictive factors and systematic review of the literature. Curr Opin Otolaryngol Head Neck Surg 2012;20(1):58–65.
11. Fairbanks DN, Fairbanks GR. Nasal septal perforation repair: 25-year experience with the flap and graft technique. Am J Cosmet Surg 1994;11:189–94.
12. Beckmann N, Ponnappan A, Campana J, et al. Posterior septal resection a simple surgical option for management of nasal septal perforation. JAMA Otolaryngol Head Neck Surg 2014;140(2):150–4.
13. Delaney SW. Evolution of the septoplasty: maximizing functional and aesthetic outcomes in nasal surgery. Mathews J Otolaryngol 2017;1(1):1–9.
14. Kridel RWH. Combined septal perforation repair with revision rhinoplasty. Facial Plast Surg Clin North Am 1995;3(4):459–72.

Correction of the Over-resected Nose

Abdul Nassimizadeh, MBChB, BMedSci, MRCS[a],
Mohammad Nassimizadeh, MBChB, BMedSci, MRCS[a], Jinli Wu, PA-C[b], Donald B. Yoo, MD[c,d,e],*

KEYWORDS

- Rhinoplasty • Revision rhinoplasty • Rib cartilage • DCF • Diced cartilage • Fascia

KEY POINTS

- Rhinoplasty traces its roots to reconstructing a nose after previous trauma, and now revision rhinoplasty shares a similar aim in restoring a nose subsequent to previous iatrogenic surgical trauma.
- Nasal anatomy should be accurately assessed for functional and aesthetic deficiencies in a both a component and holistic manner to determine the optimal treatment plan.
- Careful and accurate assessment of a patient's expectations after the physical and emotional trauma of prior surgery is paramount to a successful revision rhinoplasty result.
- Restoration of function should coincide with creation of an aesthetically balanced nose, not supersede it.

INTRODUCTION

The earliest description of rhinoplasty is found within ancient Egyptian text and dates back to 3000 BC, describing reconstructive rhinoplasty after rhinectomy for a plethora of crimes (**Figs. 1–14**).[1,2] Subsequent modifications, materials, techniques, and approach can be found internationally, often with periods of progress alongside moments of military struggles.[2] Although the aim of these rudimentary surgeries was to create the semblance of a nose, during the progression of rhinoplasty into the cosmetic domain, over the past half century, the objective has often shifted toward creating greater definition and refinement to the nose. With the intent to reduce bulk and volume in the nose, techniques emphasizing removal of bone, cartilage, and fat proliferated, with the resultant accumulation of patients suffering from the multitudinous sequelae of over-resection.

In recent years, many surgeons have placed greater emphasis on a more conservative approach, which seeks to maintain the function of the nose, in addition to creating a naturally beautiful look, compared with excessive cartilage resection.[3] Even with better understanding of the long-term effects of overly aggressive techniques, rhinoplasty continues to be one of the most complex and challenging surgical procedures, with postoperative results affecting emotional, respiratory, biobehavioral, and immunologic factors.[4] It remains a predictable conclusion that given the sheer volume of rhinoplasty surgeries being performed by surgeons of varying qualifications and skill levels, there has been a commensurate increase in the number of patients seeking revision rhinoplasty as the popularity of primary rhinoplasty grows.[5]

Disclosure Statement: This research received no specific grant from any funding agency, commercial or not-for-profit sectors.
[a] University Hospital Birmingham, 3 Pavenham Drive, Birmingham B5 7TN, UK; [b] Yoo Plastic Surgery, 120 S Spalding Drive Suite 303, Beverly Hills, CA 90212, USA; [c] Donald B. Yoo, M.D., Inc, Facial Plastic & Reconstructive Surgery, Beverly Hills, CA, USA; [d] Division of Facial Plastic and Reconstructive Surgery, Department of Otolaryngology – Head and Neck Surgery, University of Southern California, Los Angeles, CA, USA; [e] Division of Facial Plastic and Reconstructive Surgery, Department of Otolaryngology – Head and Neck Surgery, University of California – Los Angeles, Los Angeles, CA, USA
* Corresponding author. 120 South Spalding Drive, Suite 303, Beverly Hills, CA 90212.
E-mail address: info@donyoomd.com

Facial Plast Surg Clin N Am 27 (2019) 451–463
https://doi.org/10.1016/j.fsc.2019.07.003
1064-7406/19/© 2019 Elsevier Inc. All rights reserved.

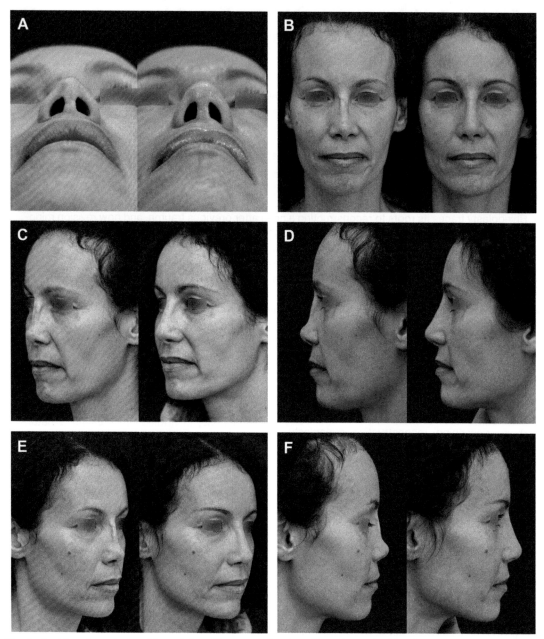

Fig. 1. Revision rhinoplasty with costal cartilage and diced cartilage fascia (DCF). (*A*) revision rhinoplasty base view. (*B*) revision rhinoplasty frontal view. (*C*) revision rhinoplasty left 3qt view. (*D*) revision rhinoplasty left profile view. (*E*) revision rhinoplasty right 3qt view. (*F*) revision rhinoplasty right profile view.

The incidence of postoperative nasal deformities requiring further surgical management approaches 20%, depending on the study, and may in actuality be far higher given most patients dissatisfied with a surgical result do not return to the original surgeon and given that no study has comprehensively evaluated the rate of patients seeking revision over a lifetime of healing.[6] By some estimates, likely conservative, over-resection accounts for approximately 26% of secondary rhinoplasty consults and is a frequent cause of patient dissatisfaction.[7-9]

In the current age of social media and emphasis on facial aesthetics, rhinoplasty continues to be a highly sought-after procedure.[4] Accordingly, the modern rhinoplasty surgeon should be versed in techniques to preserve the structural integrity of the nose, even when the objective is to create a

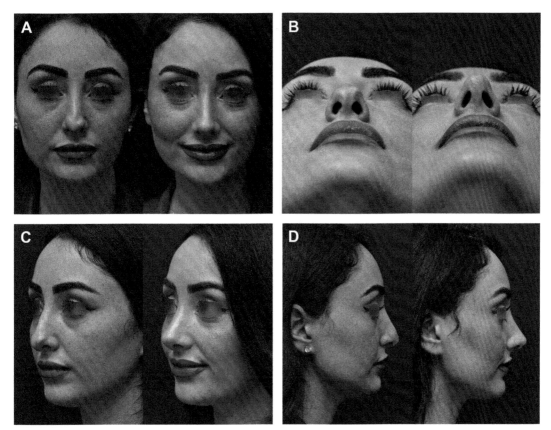

Fig. 2. Revision rhinoplasty with auricular cartilage. (*A*) revision rhinoplasty frontal view. (*B*) revision rhinoplasty base view. (*C*) primary rhinoplasty left 3qt view. (*D*) revision rhinoplasty right profile view.

smaller or more defined nose. This review considers both the issues resulting from over-resection and the techniques to effectively manage the correction of an over-reduced nose.

NASAL ANALYSIS

Meticulous nasal analysis and anatomic diagnosis are crucial when assessing a patient with over-resection. These involve a combination of detailed history taking, physical examination, and holistic analysis. A systematic approach helps to facilitate analysis and allows for comprehensive consideration of all components necessary to plan for a successful reconstructive revision rhinoplasty. Although the authors prefer an inside-out (nasal cavity to external nasal pyramid) and top-to-bottom approach (nasofrontal angle to subnasale), the important components of a systematic approach to nasal analysis are consistency and the ability to be applied efficiently to every patient.

Intranasal

Internal nasal examination assesses the septum. Some of the issues with overzealous surgery

include shortened nasal length, columellar retraction, twisting dorsal or caudal septum, saddle-nose deformity, ozena or empty nose syndrome, and septal perforation. Loss of septal height or strength from over-resection or aggressive manipulation and scoring of the septum may cause a saddle-nose deformity or deviations and deflections along the dorsal and caudal septum. At this stage, it is important to evaluate the patency of the internal and external nasal valves and the condition of the inferior turbinates.

Upper Third

The nasofrontal angle typically starts at the supratarsal crease. This point may be lower in patients with an over-resected dorsum. Presentation with a low radix accounts for a third of secondary rhinoplasty patients, with increased frequency found in men.[10] Localization of the radix can be undertaken using several methods, with normal distance to the inner canthus in the region of 6 mm. The distance between the corneal plane and the radix plane is between 9 mm and 14 mm. Ideal radix height is 0.28 of the ideal nasal length.[10,11]

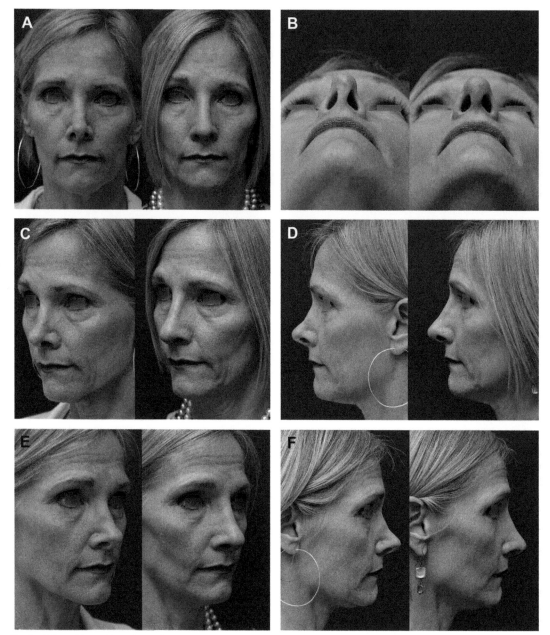

Fig. 3. (*A*) revision rhinoplasty frontal view. (*B*) revision rhinoplasty base view. (*C*) revision rhinoplasty left 3qt view. (*D*) revision rhinoplasty profile view. (*E*) revision rhinoplasty right 3qt view. (*F*) revision rhinoplasty right profile view.

The risk of a polly beak deformity is higher in patients with a deep nasofrontal angle.[12,13] This is typically found in combination with over-resection of the bony dorsum, a prominent cartilaginous dorsum, and drooping tip and accounts for almost half of revision rhinoplasty cases.[14]

The width of the bony pyramid should be assessed for asymmetry, collapse, or a subjective callous deformity. Bony vault issues often stem from asymmetric, incomplete, or overzealous osteotomy lines. With regard to subjective callous deformity, real callous deformity is rare, and most variabilities are secondary to irregularities of the nasal bone handling intraoperatively or extensive en bloc resection.[13,15]

Middle Third

The contour of the dorsum should be assessed, and any irregularity should be noted.

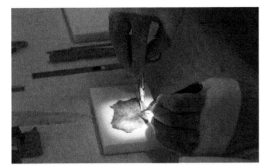

Fig. 4. Trimming of excess soft tissue from deep temporalis fascia.

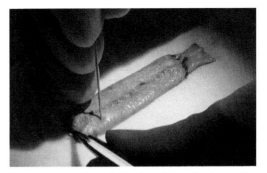

Fig. 6. Fenestration of diced cartilage fascia to allow for efflux of fluid, and to promote ingrowth.

Over-resection can result in excessive supratip break, deviation, and scooped or polly beak appearance. These can result from inadequate preoperative analysis and because of swelling, minor deviation can be difficult to recognize intraoperatively.

The upper lateral cartilages can be simultaneously affected. The angle between the septum and upper lateral cartilage is between 10° and 15°. Soft tissue structures work via a tension system, provided in conjunction with the septal cartilage. This tension is principally responsible for an even dorsal aesthetic line and air flow resistance in the middle vault.[12] Over-resection of the cartilaginous dorsal structures can result in internal nasal valve collapse, defined as narrowing of the middle vault to less than 75% of cephalic or caudal third of the nose, or an inverted-V deformity after hump reduction.[10,11,16]

Lower Third

The lower third is the most challenging aspect of successful rhinoplasty results, with effects of skin quality and thickness crucial when undergoing surgical planning. Tip projection is dependent on preservation of the alar–septum–upper lateral cartilage complex, in addition to thickness of coverage.[10,11,17]

The nasal tip is analyzed for projection and rotation. Adequacy of nasal tip projection defines when approximately 50% lies anterior to the vertically crossed lip line.[10] The lower lateral cartilages should be assessed for width, symmetry, and position. Over-resection can result in external nasal valve collapse, pinched appearance of the nasal tip, alar retraction, and loss of tip definition.

Alar rim over-reduction produces loss of natural alar flare and excessively narrow nostrils. Retraction of the alar rim secondary to over-aggressive cephalic trimming can produce excessive columella show.

The columella is assessed for increased or decreased show, with special attention placed to the columella-lobular and the columella-labial angles.

Psychological Analysis

Despite aesthetic surgery improving quality of life, self-confidence, and social interactions, body image and psychological appraisal are vital. An estimated 5% of patients presenting for cosmetic surgery are found to have body dysmorphic disorder.[18] The distinction between patients with legitimate cosmetic concerns and those with an excessive preoccupation regarding an imagined

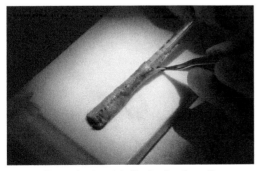

Fig. 5. Filling of DCF with finely diced cartilage.

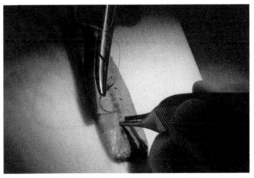

Fig. 7. Placement of corset sutures to fine-tune the size and shape of the DCF.

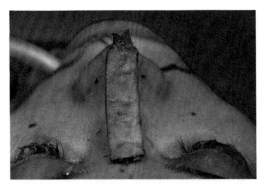

Fig. 8. Sizing DCF graft by ex vivo placment.

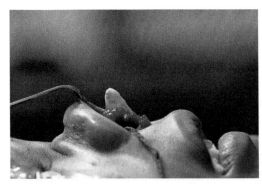

Fig. 10. Septal extension graft to establish durable tip projection and nasolabial angle.

defect of their physical appearance is a cornerstone of successful surgery.[19–21]

SURGICAL TECHNIQUES
Dorsal Augmentation

Given the relative lack of purely objective experimentation and testing in rhinoplasty, no gold standard criterion exists for dorsal augmentation. Historically, surgeons attempted augmentation using everyday materials, including ivory and jade. The ideal graft, existing only as a concept, combines biocompatibility, low complication rates, and long-term stable results.[22,23] Through the years, there have been attempts to improve outcomes using various autogenous and synthetic grafts. These have included cartilage, bone, fascia, diced cartilage and fascia, silicone, Medpore, polytetrafluorethylene, Supramid, Proplast, Vicryl, and Mersilene.[24–37]

With mild to moderate amounts of dorsal augmentation, many contemporary surgeons favor autogenous grafts in an onlay configuration.[24,28] This is secondary to excellent biotolerance, low rates of infection, extrusion, and displacement. The combination of potential drawbacks, however, including donor site morbidity, longer operating times, and larger volumes of graft materials required prompted surgeons to explore synthetic materials. Despite carrying advantages, including abundant supply, lack of second surgical site and low cost, there are inherent complications, such as high rates of mobilization, infection, and extrusion, especially in areas of tension or patients with thin skin. This drove surgeons pursue the avenue of autogenous grafts more intently.[22,23,38–44]

The senior author prefers the use of diced cartilage in a dorsal augmentation in this scenario. This has been periodically documented in literature as early as 1943 by Peer and 1951 by Cottle but did not gain contemporary widespread acceptance at the time.[45–47] Modifications of the concept of using diced cartilage as the building block for dorsal augmentation have been variously described, primarily adding assorted tissue adhesives to ease shaping of the graft, altering the material wrapping the cartilage, or foregoing encasement altogether.[48–52] Previous attempts with Surgicel wrapping, however, encountered frequent absorption rates, and the use of synthetic porcine mesothelium–wrapped diced cartilage was associated with lower cartilage viability, despite the elimination of harvesting fascia.[53,54]

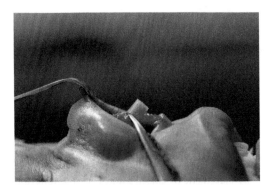

Fig. 9. Extended spreader grafts.

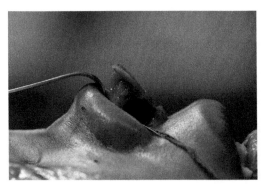

Fig. 11. Shield graft.

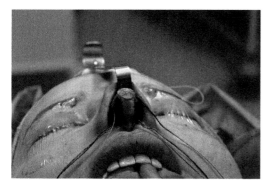

Fig. 12. Tip-refining grafts.

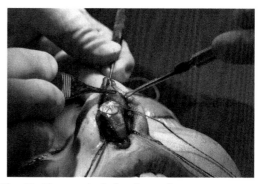

Fig. 14. Placement of alar rim graft.

Diced cartilage with fascia represents a potentially ideal graft for augmentation of the dorsum, because it makes use of the lower complication rates associated with autogenous grafts while providing a graft that has the ability to recreate dorsal aesthetic lines in a natural and predictable manner.

Cartilage may be harvested from the septum, ears, or rib, depending on the volume requirements of the dorsal augmentation. The physical characteristics of the cartilage sources vary significantly and have an impact on surgical outcomes. Auricular cartilage is pliable and easily shaped. The cymba concha, due its curvature, is suitable for reconstruction of the lateral crura, whereas the cavum concha is thicker and stiffer, making it better placed for nasal tip work.[38] Patients with major deformities that require an increase of the nasal dorsum by greater than 4 mm, however, suffer poorer results with auricular grafts. In this scenario, costal cartilage provides significantly larger volume for extensive work.[22]

The senior author advocates dicing of the costal cartilage to less than 0.5-mm pieces to minimize the risk of contour irregularities. Fascia may be obtained from multiple sources, but temporalis fascia is the thinnest of commonly used options and

produces minimal donor site morbidity. Care should be taken in fascia harvest to ensure adequate surface area (>5 cm × 3.5 cm) and that all extraneous fat and muscle is meticulously removed from the fascia to create the thinnest and most uniform layer of tissue. After this, it is sutured longitudinally into a cylindrical shape, uniquely sized to each patient. One end of the fascia is closed and subsequently filled with an estimated volume of cartilage, before being placed along the nasal dorsum. The diced cartilage fascia (DCF) does contract and dehydrate when healed, so every effort is made to remove fluid prior to making measurements for its final dimensions.

A needle is used to create fenestrations throughout the DCF, to allow for free effusion of any remaining fluid from within the construct and to promote quicker fibrous and vascular ingrowth into the graft. Once healed, the diced cartilage within the DCF provides the lasting volume, while the fascia simply acts as a temporary vehicle to place and shape the cartilage. Corset sutures are placed to taper the graft from a cylindrical shape to a more parabolic shape, consistent with the appearance of the desired dorsal aesthetic lines. The DCF is secured along its cephalic and caudal ends and its body shaped by casting. A percutaneous suture is placed through the marked starting point, and secured to the cephalic end of DCF.

Depressed Nasal Bones

Overzealous or asymmetric osteotomies leading to unilateral or bilateral depressed nasal walls are often difficult to treat. This is encountered more typically after composite reduction of the nasal dorsum en block, which is found to be more difficult to control and leaves little room for error.[3] Component rhinoplasty, addressing each section of the nasal dorsum individually, seems to be a more logical option in resections of greater than 2 mm. There also has been the introduction of a smaller osteotome with the aim of producing a

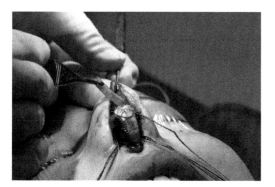

Fig. 13. Rim graft.

more controlled and less traumatic method, but there have been noted issues with the probability of relapsing of the in-fractured bones to the preoperative position.[55,56]

It is important to consider whether the excessive narrowing of nasal bones has caused any functional issues. In revision cases, options include reosteotomy; spreader grafts or augmentation of the depressed side wall with fascia, such as temporalis fascia; cartilage; or a synthetic graft as camouflage.[15]

The use of spreader grafts extended cephalad and reosteotomy can aid the placement of the dorsal graft, with a wider base for stability improving overall cosmesis.[57] There has also been a description of lifting the nasal bones into the desired position with forceps and making appropriately placed holes in the bones for the placement of either sutures or wire.[56,58]

Middle Vault Collapse

Despite the availability of techniques, none has been as singularly accepted as the spreader graft, introduced in 1984. Although initially conceived to reconstruct the middle vault in patients with short nasal bones, it was soon identified as having the additional benefit of support for the lateral nasal wall.[59] At first, this was applied after dorsal hump reduction to reinforce the upper lateral cartilages and prevent their collapse against the septum. Since then, the technique has been widely adopted for a variety of functional cosmetic indications, including correction of internal nasal valve collapse; bridging a long, narrow middle vault in patients with short nasal bones; correcting lack of dorsal support of the lateral nasal walls; widening the middle third of the nose; straightening or stabilization of a high dorsally deviated septum; creating straight dorsal aesthetic lines; and lengthening a short nose as a caudal extension graft.[60]

The open rhinoplasty approach for the placement of spreader grafts is used more commonly because it has the advantages of improved visualization and potentially more accurate fixation. Spreader grafts placed in this manner are almost uniformly secured with sutures.

Middle vault collapse can affect both nasal aesthetic and function. A narrowed middle vault constitutes an angle less than 10° to 15° between the dorsal septum and the upper lateral cartilage.[10] Literature highlights that middle vault collapse and narrowing in primary rhinoplasty is approximately 4 times more common than obstruction secondary to nasal septal deviation.[10,61] Performing a Cottle test preoperatively

highlights or delineates the requirement intraoperatively. Treatment typically involves the use of a dorsal onlay graft orunilateral or bilateral spreader grafts with suture fixation between the upper lateral cartilage and septum. These are usually paired, longitudinal grafts. Other alternatives described include placing the graft in mucoperichondrial pockets with no suture fixation.[38] The graft acts to widen the nasal valve angle, and it is found to be the most successful management option in correcting middle vault deformity or nasal valve related airway problems.[62]

The length and shape of the spreader grafts may vary. The grafts may extend above the level of the dorsum to slightly augment the dorsum or extend caudally beyond the septal angle to lengthen the nose.

Septal Augmentation

If septal work is required in secondary rhinoplasty, it may be approached either through a transfixion incision or from above after the upper lateral cartilages have been released. Typically, care is taken to preserve the L-strut. The recommendation regarding amount of L-strut required varies among surgeons, with values ranging between 5 mm and 15 mm.[63] The integrity and strength of the septal L-strut can be compromised, however, in previous rhinoplasty. In these scenarios, dorsal spreader grafts may be utilized to provide support and stabilization bilaterally. Other surgeons advocate the use of bone from the bony septum and multiple drilled holes for suturing, which in turn increases stability in the deviated septum. There is the belief that a strong support network is required to resist the memory effect of a curved septum and prevent recurrence.[38,64] Similarly, if there is dislocation off the maxillary crest, appropriate repositioning is crucial. To check stability intraoperatively, the vertical stability and horizontal stability tests should be performed by grasping the caudal septum with forceps and maneuvering both vertically and horizontally. Different suturing techniques have been advocated in this scenario to improve stability, including mattress, Byrd, or Mustard suture techniques.[65-69]

In some cases, there is loss of tip support and projection secondary to septal over-resection. Correction can include the use of septal extension or extended spreader grafts. Having been first introduced in 1998, these require the presence of a stable caudal septum and are sutured to the septal angle, with the aim of extending into the tip lobule complex. At least 3 mm to 4 mm of the caudal septum and the graft must overlap for adequate superior and inferior suture fixation.[70]

The results of a singular cartilage graft for extension depend on the condition of the harvested graft. There is the possibility when using septal or auricular cartilage that there is already some bending even without a history of trauma, and as a result the senior author advocates the use of a bilateral extension type of graft typically utilizing costal cartilage.[65,71] Typically, the central cartilage slice is trimmed to approximately 2 mm with the flat region used for a septal extension graft. Because the alar cartilage is connected to surrounding ligamentous structures, sufficient release is required to allow for appropriate reconstruction. If performed appropriately, there is the potential to add length while controlling the nasal tip bidirectionally and 3-D.[63]

The mucosa and perichondrium form the composite layer of mucoperichondrium of the septum. Dissection through this plane can inadvertently happen during overzealous surgery. Resultant mucosal thinning, hematoma formation, and septal perforation are all known consequences. With the perichondrial layer known to aid biomechanical strength and other known issues with septal perforations, it is imperative to reconstruct these issues in secondary surgery.[72] This can be addressed with either extensive undermining of remaining tissue; mobilization of regional flaps, such as septal mucoperichondrial flap in smaller defects; or pedicled flaps, including a gingivobuccal flap.

Alar Augmentation

Lateral crural augmentation depends on the quantity of cartilage present in the tip and available cartilage for grafting. The projection and the tip can be considered through Anderson tripod mechanism, consisting of the 2 lateral and conjoined medial crura.[73] If the angle of cephalic divergence is greater than 45°, there is significant alar cartilage malpositioning.[10] In scenarios where there is alar retraction, alar rim collapse, or malpositioned but present lateral crura, lateral crural strut grafts may be used. These can re-establish stability in collapsed or concave lateral crura, ultimately improving shape. Cartilage grafts are placed between the skin and lateral crus, before being sutured into adequate position. They end within a pocket inferior to the alar groove and lateral to the piriform aperture, to reduce the appearance of a bulge superiorly to the ala and improve nasal airflow simultaneously. Some surgeons advocate the use of solely resection and relocation of the lateral crura; however, the authors believe this increases the risk of postoperative deformity without stabilizing cartilage.[16] With regard to cartilage, it is important to fashion 1-mm slices to avoid excessive external protrusion or irregularities. Other lateral crura augmentation surgical strategies include lateral cural steal and overlay techniques.[74]

In rare scenarios where there is absent or unusable medial and lateral crura, the caudal leg of the tripod must be initially reconstructed prior to use of lateral strut grafts. These must be shaped appropriately to mimic acceptably the contour of both the medial and lateral portions. To avoid irregularities, an onlay graft consisting of fascia or perichondrium is utilized to act as camouflage. This requires both extensive understanding of anatomic framework and large quantity of cartilage, which is only available from the rib.

Alar rim retraction specifically can occur after overaggressive cephalic trim. It is normally advocated to retain at least a 6-mm alar strip and carefully resect the vestibular mucosa if required. In scenarios of unilateral asymmetry or bilateral retraction, there is the potential of using only alar batten or alar rim grafts.

Alar batten and rim grafts were first introduced in 1997 and have steadily increased in use internationally, with the idea of improving structural integrity and preventing collapse during negative upper airway pressure rather than increase cross-sectional area.[75–77] Preoperatively, nasal strips act as a positive predictor of patients who could potentially benefit from alar batten grafts. There are even suggestions that a majority of patients who undergo rhinoplasty benefitting from some sort of graft around the alar.[77]

Tip Refining

Re-establishing tip support and projection can be challenging in secondary rhinoplasty, with nasal tip projection the most frequent postoperative deformity.[78] A columella strut graft can significantly aid this process. Advantages similarly include stabilization of the caudal edge, which acts as a resistor to contraction from scar tissue or swelling.[59] Due to a combination of delicacy and required rigidity of the area, auricular and septal cartilage can at times be insufficient because of their inherent properties. Initially a pocket must be created by dissecting between the medial crura appropriately, prior to placement of an adequately sized graft for the patient. The importance is underlined in the literature, with columella strut placement providing permanent results for tip projection and protection independent of the nasal septum and other techniques.[12,79] This structural integrity is typically lost with an endonasal technique both clinically and in specimen-based studies.[80,81]

When the strength or resiliency of the lower lateral cartilages is lacking, rigid tip support is preferred by the senior author because it allows precise and enduring establishment of both nasal tip projection and rotation. Although it does sacrifice the natural flexibility of the nasal tip, in cases of revision rhinoplasty without adequate support from the lower lateral cartilages, this becomes a necessary compromise. The preferred method of fixation is in-line with the caudal septum and secured between extended spreader grafts. In this application for the over-resected nose, a stable platform may be re-established for placement of a dorsal onlay graft, while also lengthening the nose and increasing projection of the nasal tip.

In 1989, the systematic nondestructive approach to nasal tip suturing was introduced and the tip rotation suture at a later date by the same author.[82] In 1997 and 1998, further modifications were made, but despite these methods there were still numerous patients with postoperative change and tip rotation.[83,84] Other techniques include scoring, crushing, and resection of local anatomy. Tip grafts are designed to enhance the nasal tip profile or change definition or projection. Projection refers to the posterior-anterior distance or the distance from the subnasal to the tip-defining point as seen on the profile view.[84,85] Tip grafts provide an ideal tool due to disruption of the supporting structures around the tip during rhinoplasty.

The accuracy and eventual quality of tip refining surgery are dependent on thorough preoperative assessment. These are especially useful when attempting to address scarred or thick skin.[86,87] The strong shield graft is tapered for accurate placement, which can vary from integration to high placement depending on desired results.[86] If placed superior to the ala, a cap graft must be added to avoid external irregularities, and multiple grafts may be required in the over-resected nose. In patients with thin or fragile skin, it may be useful to consider concomitant fascia as a form of camouflage.

SUMMARY

Over-reduction of the nose during rhinoplasty occurs routinely, but fortunately there are reliable and predictable methods of addressing many of the issues arising from over-aggressive rhinoplasty. The contemporary rhinoplasty surgeon should seek to preserve the structural integrity of the nose during primary cases, while becoming facile in the analysis, approach, and execution of techniques to reconstruct and restore the over-reduced nose. Refinements in revision rhinoplasty techniques have brought about increasingly safer, more consistent, and durable results, although the persistent challenge for rhinoplasty surgeons moving forward remains to create even more aesthetically attractive noses in the midst of previous trauma.

REFERENCES

1. Shiffman MA, Giuseppe DA. Cosmetic surgery: art and techniques. In: Shiffman MA, Giuseppe DA, editors. History of cosmetic surgery. New York: Springer Heidelberg; 2013. p. 20–1.
2. Rinzler CA, Grant RT, Darrow S. In the encyclopedia of cosmetic and plastic surgery. New York: Facts on File, Inc. An imprint of Infobase Publishing; 2009. p. 151–2.
3. Mohmand MH, Ahmad M. Component rhinoplasty. World J Plast Surg 2014;3(1):18–23.
4. Crosara PF, Nunes FB, Rodrigues DS, et al. Rhinoplasty complications and reoperations: systematic review. Int Arch Otorhinolaryngol 2017;21(1): 97–101.
5. Kang IG, Kim ST, Lee SH, et al. Failed septal extension graft in a patient with a history of radiotherapy. Maxillofac Plast Reconstr Surg 2016;38(1):40.
6. Rees TD, Krupp S, Wood-Smith D. Secondary rhinoplasty. Plast Reconstr Surg 1970;46:332.
7. Nassab R, Matti B. Presenting concerns and surgical management of secondary rhinoplasty. Aesthet Surg J 2015;35(2):137–44.
8. Sykes JM. Management of the middle nasal third in revision rhinoplasty. Facial Plast Surg 2008;24(3): 339–47.
9. Sandel HD 4th, Perkins SW. Management of the short nose deformity in revision rhinoplasty. Facial Plast Surg 2008;24(3):310–26.
10. Eskandarlou M, Motamed S. Evaluation of frequency of four common nasal anatomical deformities in primary rhinoplasty in a tehran plastic surgery center. World J Plast Surg 2014;3(2):122–8.
11. Gunter JP, Robrich RJ, Adams WP. Nasal surgery by the masters. 2nd edition. Dallas (TX): Quality Medical Publishing; 2007. p. 135–40.
12. Rettinger G. Risks and complications in rhinoplasty. GMS Curr Top Otorhinolaryngol Head Neck Surg 2008;6:Doc08.
13. Constantian MB. Four common anatomic variants that predispose to unfavorable rhinoplasty results: a study based on 150 consecutive secondary rhinoplasties. Plast Reconstr Surg 2000;105(1):316–31.
14. Tardy ME Jr, Kron TK, Younger R, et al. The cartilaginous pollybeak: etiology, prevention and treatment. Facial Plast Surg 1989;6(2):113–20.

15. Gubisch W, Dacho A. Aesthetic rhinoplasty plus brow, eyelid and conchal surgery: pitfalls - complications - prevention. GMS Curr Top Otorhinolaryngol Head Neck Surg 2013;12:Doc07.

16. Constantian MB. Rhinoplasty craft and magic. 2nd edition. St Louis (MO): Quality Medical Publishing; 2009. p. 187–250.

17. Pitanguy I, Salgado F, Radwanski HN, et al. The surgical importance of the dermocartilaginous ligament of the nose. Plast Reconstr Surg 1995;95(5): 790–4.

18. Cochran CS, Gunter JP. Secondary rhinoplasty and the use of autogenous rib cartilage grafts. Clin Plast Surg 2010;37(2):371–82.

19. Picavet VA, Prokopakis EP, Gabriëls L, et al. High prevalence of body dysmorphic disorder symptoms in patients seeking rhinoplasty. Plast Reconstr Surg 2011;128(2):509–17.

20. Veale D, Ellison N, Werner TG, et al. Development of a cosmetic procedure screening questionnaire (COPS) for body dysmorphic disorder. J Plast Reconstr Aesthet Surg 2012;65(4):530–2.

21. Rohrich RJ, Muzaffar AR. Primary rhinoplasty. In: Guyuron B, editor. Plastic surgery: indications, operations, and outcomes. St Louis (MO): Mosby; 2000. p. 2631–45.

22. Alvarez-Buylla Blanco M, Sarandeses García A, Chao Vieites J, et al. Functional and aesthetic results after augmentation rhinoplasty. Acta Otorrinolaringol Esp 2011;62(5):347–54.

23. Immerman S, White W, Constantinides M. Cartilage grafting in nasal reconstruction. Facial Plast Surg Clin North Am 2011;19:175–82.

24. Krause CJ. Augmentation rhinoplasty. Otolaryngol Clin North Am 1975;8:743–52.

25. Wheeler ES, Kawamoto HK, Zarem HA. Bone grafts for nasal reconstruction. Plast Reconstr Surg 1982; 69:9–18.

26. Romo T 3rd, Jablonski RD. Nasal reconstruction using split calvarial grafts. Otolaryngol Head Neck Surg 1992;107:622–30.

27. Leaf N. SMAS autografts for the nasal dorsum. Plast Reconstr Surg 1996;97:1249–52.

28. Regnault P. Nasal augmentation in the problem nose. Aesthetic Plast Surg 1987;11:1–5.

29. Khoo BC. Augmentation rhinoplasty in the orientals. Plast Reconstr Surg 1964;34:81–8.

30. Beekhuis GJ. Silastic alar-columellar prosthesis in conjunction with rhinoplasty. Arch Otolaryngol 1982;108:429–32.

31. Wellisz T. Clinical experience with the Medpor porous polyethylene implant. Aesthetic Plast Surg 1993;17:339–44.

32. Godin MS, Waldman SR, Johnson CM Jr. The use of expanded polytetrafluoroethylene (Gore-Tex) in rhinoplasty. A 6-year experience. Arch Otolaryngol Head Neck Surg 1995;121:1131–6.

33. Queen TA, Palmer FR 3rd. Gore-Tex for nasal augmentation: a recent series and a review of the literature. Ann Otol Rhinol Laryngol 1995;104:850–2.

34. Adams JS. Grafts and implants in nasal and chin augmentation. A rational approach to material selection. Otolaryngol Clin North Am 1987;20: 913–30.

35. Gilmore J. Use of Vicryl mesh in prevention of post-rhinoplasty dorsal irregularities. Ann Plast Surg 1989;22:105–7.

36. Juraha LZ. Experience with alternative material for nasal augmentation. Aesthetic Plast Surg 1992;16: 133–40.

37. Fanous N. Mersilene tip implants in rhinoplasty: a review of 98 cases. Plast Reconstr Surg 1991;87: 662–71.

38. Gendeh BS. Clinical study of graft selection in malaysian rhinoplasty patients. ISRN Otolaryngol 2013;2013:639643.

39. Sertel S, Venara-Vulpe II, Pasche P. Correction of severe columella and tip retraction in silicone implanted Asian short noses. J Otolaryngol Head Neck Surg 2016;45:19.

40. Lee MJ, Song HM. Asian rhinoplasty with rib cartilage. Semin Plast Surg 2015;29(4):262–8.

41. Farrior RT, Farrior EH, Cook R. Special rhinoplasty techniques. In: Cummings CW, Flint PW, Harker LA, et al, editors. Cummings: otolarynglogy head neck surgery. 4th edition. Philadelphia: Elsevier Mosby; 2005. p. 1078–114.

42. Kreymerman PA, Fardo D. Rhinoplasty augmentation: treatment. Plastic Surg 2008;25:236–42.

43. Araco A, Gravante G, Araco F, et al. Autologous cartilage graft rhinoplasties. Aesthetic Plast Surg 2006;30:169–74.

44. Sclafani AP. Nasal implants: treatment. Otolaryngol Facial Plastic Surg 2008;12:224–8.

45. Burian F. The plastic surgery atlas. New York: Macmillan; 1968.

46. Peer LA. Diced cartilage grafts. Arch Otolaryngol 1943;38:156–65.

47. Cottle MH. Nasal surgery in children. Eye Ear Nose Throat Mon 1951;30:32–8.

48. Berghaus A, San Nicoló M, Jacobi C. Use of a fibrinogen-thrombin sponge in rhinoplasty. HNO 2018;66(2):103–10.

49. Cerkes N, Basaran K. Diced cartilage grafts wrapped in rectus abdominis fascia for nasal dorsum augmentation. Plast Reconstr Surg 2016;137(1): 43–51.

50. Hoehne J, Gubisch W, Kreutzer C, et al. Refining the nasal dorsum with free diced cartilage. Facial Plast Surg 2016;32(4):345–50.

51. Erol OO. Injection of compressed diced cartilage in the correction of secondary and primary rhinoplasty: a new technique with 12 years' experience. Plast Reconstr Surg 2017;140(5):673e–85e.

52. Tasman AJ. Advances in nasal dorsal augmentation with diced cartilage. Curr Opin Otolaryngol Head Neck Surg 2013;21(4):365–71.

53. Correia-Sá I, Amarante J, Horta R, et al. Secondary rhinoplasty using the technique of Turkish Delight: a case report and a brief review of the literature. Acta Med Port 2015;28(1):122–6.

54. Bramos A, Perrault DP, Fedenko AN, et al. Porcine mesothelium-wrapped diced cartilage grafts for nasal reconstruction. Tissue Eng A 2018;24(7–8): 672–81.

55. Erişir F, Tahamiler R. Lateral osteotomies in rhinoplasty: a safer and less traumatic method. Aesthet Surg J 2008;28(5):518–20.

56. Bali ZU, Sır E, Ahmedov A, et al. A novel method to prevent complications of nasal osteotomy: matress suture which traverses lateral walls and septum. Kulak Burun Bogaz Ihtis Derg 2015; 25(6):324–8.

57. Gunter JP, Cochran CS, Marin VP. Dorsal augmentation with autogenous rib cartilage. Semin Plast Surg 2008;22(2):74–89.

58. Tebbetts JB. Osteotomies. In: Tebbetts JB, editor. Primer rhinoplasty. 2nd edition. (TX): Mosby; 2008. p. 211–45.

59. Sheen JH. Spreader graft: a method of reconstructing the roof of the middle nasal vault following rhinoplasty. Plast Reconstr Surg 1984; 73(2):230–9.

60. Yoo DB, Jen A, et al. Endonasal placement of spreader grafts. Experience in 41 Consecutive patients. Arch Facial Plast Surg 2012;14(5): 318–22.

61. Constantian MB. The two essential elements for planning tip surgery in primary and secondary rhinoplasty. Observations based on review of 100 consecutive patients. Plast Reconstr Surg 2004; 114:1571–81.

62. Acarturk S, Arslan E, Demirkan F, et al. An algorithm for deciding alternative grafting materials used in secondary rhinoplasty. J Plast Reconstr Aesthet Surg 2006;59(4):409–16.

63. Jeong JY. Obtaining maximal stability with a septal extension technique in East asian rhinoplasty. Arch Plast Surg 2014;41(1):19–28.

64. Gendeh BS, Tan VES. Open septorhinoplasty: operative technique and grafts. Med J Malaysia 2007; 62(1):13–8.

65. Hubbard TJ. Exploiting the septum for maximal tip control. Ann Plast Surg 2000;44:173–80.

66. Oh SH, Kang NH, Woo JS, et al. Stabilization of unilateral septal extension graft using pivot locking Suture. J Korean Soc Aesthetic Plast Surg 2008;14: 156–60.

67. Gruber RP, Nahai F, Bogdan MA, et al. Changing the convexity and concavity of nasal cartilages and cartilage grafts with horizontal mattress sutures:

part I. Experimental results. Plast Reconstr Surg 2005;115:589–94.

68. Gruber RP, Nahai F, Bogdan MA, et al. Changing the convexity and concavity of nasal cartilages and cartilage grafts with horizontal mattress sutures: part II. Clinical results. Plast Reconstr Surg 2005; 115:595–606.

69. Calderón-Cuéllar LT, Trujillo-Hernandez B, Vasquez C, et al. Modified mattress suture technique to correct anterior septal deviation. Plast Reconstr Surg 2004;114:1436–41.

70. Toriumi DM. New concepts in nasal tip contouring. Arch Facial Plast Surg 2006;8:156–85.

71. Byrd HS, Salomon J, Flood J. Correction of the crooked nose. Plast Reconstr Surg 1998;102: 2148–57.

72. Kim DW, Egan KK, O'Grady K, et al. Biomechanical strength of human nasal septal lining: comparison of the constituent layers. Laryngoscope 2005;115: 1451–3.

73. Hoffmann JF. Management of the twisted nose. Oper Tech Otolayngol Head Neck Surg 1999; 10(3):232–7.

74. Foda HM, Kridel RW. Lateral crural steal and lateral crural overlay: an objective evaluation. Arch Otolaryngol Head Neck Surg 1999;125(12): 1365–70.

75. Bewick JC, Buchanan MA, Frosh AC. Internal nasal valve incompetence is effectively treated using batten graft functional rhinoplasty. Int J Otolaryngol 2013;2013:734795.

76. Toriumi DM, Josen J, Weinberger M, et al. Use of alar batten grafts for correction of nasal valve collapse. Arch Otolaryngol Head Neck Surg 1997; 123(8):802–8.

77. Guyuron B, Bigdeli Y, Sajjadian A. Dynamics of the alar rim graft. Plast Reconstr Surg 2015;135(4): 981–6.

78. Tardy ME Jr, Cheng EY, Jernstrom V. Misadventures in nasal tip surgery: analysis and repair. Otolaryngol Clin North Am 1987;20(4):797–823.

79. Vuyk HD, Oakenfull C, Plaat RE. A quantitative appraisal of change in nasal tip projection after open rhinoplasty. Rhinology 1997;35:124–8.

80. Beaty MM, Dyer WK, Shawl MW. The quantification of surgical changes in nasal tip support. Arch Facial Plast Surg 2002;4(2):82–91.

81. Adams WP, Rohrich RJ, Hollier LH, et al. Anatomic basis and clinical implications for nasal tip support in open versus closed rhinoplasty. Plast Reconstr Surg 1999;103(1):255–61.

82. Tebbetts JB. Rethinking the logic and techniques of primary tip rhinoplasty: a perspective of the evolution of surgery of the nasal Tip. Otolaryngol Clin North Am 1999;32(4):741–54.

83. Guyuron B. Footplates of the medial crura. Plast Reconstr Surg 1998;101:1359–63.

84. Motamed S, Otaghvar HA, Niazi F, et al. Introducing a favourite tip definition and projection with tripod suture in rhinoplasty. J Clin Diagn Res 2017;11(1): PC05–7.

85. Simons RL, Behmand RA. Nasal tip projection, ptosis, and supratip thickening. Ear Nose Throat J 1982;61:452–5.

86. Daniel RK. Mastering in rhinoplasty: a comprehensive atlas of surgical techniques with integrated video clips. 2nd edition. Berlin: Springer; 2010.

87. Bussi M, Palonta F, Toma S. Grafting in revision rhinoplasty. Acta Otorhinolaryngol Ital 2013;33(3): 183–9.

Management of Postsurgical Empty Nose Syndrome

Jason Talmadge, MD[a], Jayakar V. Nayak, MD, PhD[b], William Yao, MD[a],
Martin J. Citardi, MD[c],*

KEYWORDS

- Empty nose syndrome • Atrophic rhinitis • Turbinate • Cotton test • ENS6Q • Nasal airway
- Upper airway

KEY POINTS

- Empty nose syndrome is considered an iatrogenic condition most often associated with excessive resection and/or compromised wound healing of the nasal turbinate tissue after surgery for nasal obstruction.
- Empty nose syndrome is a clinical diagnosis whose hallmark feature is a widely patent nasal cavity in a patient complaining of persistent nasal obstruction.
- Empty nose syndrome often presents with secondary nasal complaints and referred pain complaints that contribute to a global sense of panic, anxiety and depression.
- The Empty Nose Syndrome 6-item Questionnaire and the cotton test can help verify the diagnosis and assist with treatment planning.
- Medical treatment for empty nose syndrome includes aggressive moisturization and humidification and cognitive-behavioral and supportive therapies. Surgical approaches include replacement of turbinate tissue volume/bulk at sites of tissue loss.

INTRODUCTION

The inferior turbinate has been viewed as a prominent cause for nasal obstruction since the mid-19th century, when surgeons first described procedures designed to reduce the inferior turbinate dimensions. Initially, surgery directed at the inferior turbinate was performed using thermal and chemical coagulation techniques, but during the 20th century, inferior turbinate surgery evolved

significantly. More aggressive tissue removal to increase nasal airway patency characterized various turbinate resection procedures, with the most extensive surgery being complete inferior turbinate excision/radical turbinectomy. During 1900 to 1910, the more conservative technique of submucous resection was developed as an alternative to turbinate excision.[1] By the mid-20th century, complications such as atrophic rhinitis, turbinate

Disclosure Statement: M.J. Citardi serves as a consultant for Acclarent (Irvine, CA), Intersect ENT (Palo Alto, CA), Medical Metrics (Houston, TX), and Stryker (Kalamazoo, MI). W. Yao is a member of the Optinose (Yardley, PA) speaker's bureau. J.V. Nayak is a consultant for Medtronic (Jacksonville, FL), Olympus America (Center Valley, PA), and Cook Medical (Bloomfield, IN). He is on the scientific advisory board of Hydravascular, Inc (Milpitas, CA).The rest of the authors have nothing to disclose.
 a Department of Otolaryngology, Medical College of Wisconsin, 3400 Market Lane, Kenosha, WI 53144, USA; b Department of Otolaryngology, Stanford University School of Medicine, 801 Welch Road, Stanford, CA 94305, USA; c Department of Otorrhinolaryngology, The University of Texas Health Science Center at Houston, McGovern Medical School, 6431 Fannin Street, MSB 5.036, Houston, TX 77030, USA
* Corresponding author.
E-mail address: martin.j.citardi@uth.tmc.edu

Facial Plast Surg Clin N Am 27 (2019) 465–475
https://doi.org/10.1016/j.fsc.2019.07.005

hemorrhage, and increased nasal pain were newly reported, and many were associated with aggressive resection of inferior turbinate tissue (**Fig. 1**). As a result, many surgeons started to advocate for decreasing the volume and extent of turbinate tissue removal. Nonetheless, some surgeons continued to practice complete or near-complete turbinate resection, in the quest for maximal opening of the nasal airway, and presumably perceived patient satisfaction. Over subsequent decades, surgeons observed subtle patterns of delayed complications associated with turbinate resection, but the signs and symptoms were not formally described as a distinct clinical entity until the mid-1990s when Stenkvist and Kern coined the term empty nose syndrome (ENS).[1,2] Since then, this term has come to describe the constellation of patient complaints, physical findings, and other morbidities that are associated with aggressive turbinate resection.

Radical loss of inferior turbinate tissue (and to a lesser degree middle turbinate tissue) has been associated with the development of ENS.[3,4] Although a few surgeons have reported case series in which ENS did not develop among patients who underwent turbinate excision,[5,6] many surgeons today are increasingly aware of compelling data that support the hypothesis that changes in airflow dynamics and neurophysiology after overexcision of turbinate tissue can lead to ENS in some patients.[3,4,7–9] In recent years, clinical researchers have focused on better understanding of the diagnosis and pathophysiology of this poorly understood entity; this knowledge serves

as the foundation for improved medical and surgical treatments for ENS, as well as advocacy for mucosal-sparing surgery.[3,7,10–12]

PATHOPHYSIOLOGY OF EMPTY NOSE SYNDROME

Each inferior turbinate functions to regulate the volume, rate and quality of air passing through the nose. Turbinates also "condition" inspired air to body warmth and humidity, and trap environmental particles and pollutants.[1,13] The net effect is to provide some degree of airway resistance and sensation regarding the adequacy of nasal airflow; that is, patients will report the presence or absence of symptoms of nasal congestion, obstruction, and dryness in ways that in large part reflect inferior turbinate size and function. Obviously, reduction or resection of any portion of inferior turbinate tissue may directly impair its function or disrupt the interplay between these dynamic upper airway parameters. In the setting of complete or near-complete resection of inferior turbinate tissues, there can be disproportional loss of the beneficial effects of normal turbinate function.[4] When this happens, symptoms of ENS may develop via a number of mechanisms, including altered intranasal airflow patterns, decreased nasal resistance, impaired sense of nasal temperature regulation, and distorted nasal sensation. It should be noted that not all patients will experience these debilitating symptoms, and many patients may in fact be quite pleased with their less obstructed, patent nasal airway. The latter finding highlights both the subjective, variable nature of nasal breathing metrics between individuals, and the difficulties with establishing formal diagnostic parameters for ENS as a disease entity.

Computational fluid dynamics based on sinus computed tomography scans and MRI has emerged as a technology to study and model upper airway airflow dynamics at steady state and after procedures, including radical turbinate surgery. In the normal nasal cavity, the airflow is turbulent, and in a pattern composed of medium velocity vectors that are evenly distributed between the inferior and middle turbinates and their respective meatuses.[14–16] However, after inferior turbinate resection, there are 3 consistent shifts seen in patients suffering from ENS (as defined by the Empty Nose Syndrome 6-item Questionnaire [ENS6Q] score of >11; ENS6Q further described elsewhere in this article): (1) laminar (rather than turbulent) air flow patterns, (2) increased velocity (rather than medium velocity) airflow vectors, and (3) compromised airflow to the inferior portion of the nasal

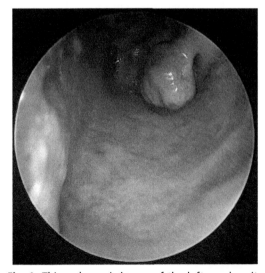

Fig. 1. This endoscopic image of the left nasal cavity demonstrates the near-complete resection of the inferior turbinate.

cavity, which shifts the airflow upward into the region of the middle meatus and the nasopharynx. These changes can potentially lead to postprocedural nasal dysfunction—perceived as suffocation, nasal dryness, and discomfort from these newly affected areas and airflow patterns.[14–16] In addition, the loss of balanced airflow distribution likely hinders the broad mucosal contact necessary for sensing airway resistance and providing conditioning functions to warm and humidify inhaled air before entering the lower airway.

Another factor is the ability of the nose to sense cool mucosal temperatures, which partly depends on the function of the receptor known as transient receptor potential cation channel subfamily M member 8 (TRPM8) within the nasal mucosa.[16,17] TRPM8 senses changes in membrane rigidity after rapid airflow and liquid evaporation; this afferent signal, transmitted to the brain via the trigeminal nerve branches, is cognitively interpreted as nasal coolness.[9] Studies have shown that the perception of nasal coolness is a prominent factor in the sensation of nasal airflow.[18] This receptor can be directly stimulated by aerosolized menthol solutions, leading to a sensation of nasal coolness without actual temperature or airway dimension changes.[17] Studies that rely on this effect of TRPM8 have confirmed the impairment or loss of this sensory mechanism in patients with ENS.[16] It has been speculated that the ability to detect mucosal cooling via the trigeminal nerve reflects the patency of the nasal passageways (and by extension the rate of airflow). Similarly, TRPM8-mediated mechanisms may also directly stimulate the limbic centers of the brain to impact pulmonary physiology.[9,19] Thus, turbinate tissue excision, which leads to loss of tissue receptors, decrease the capacity of the nose to sense coolness (and airflow) in affected patients with ENS.

Disturbance in nasal sensation after surgery has also been suggested to play a role in ENS. The inappropriate postoperative regeneration of sensorineural connections at the operative site may lead to both loss of airway sensation, as well as abnormally heightened pain responses. It is hypothesized that the damaged nerve fibers regenerate aberrant neural connections that create the sensation of pain independent of noxious stimuli. This phenomenon may be similar to Frey's syndrome, in which parasympathetic fibers reconnect with severed sympathetic nerve fibers to produce gustatory sweating after parotid surgery or to persistent skin anesthesia after head and neck incisions owing to failure of appropriate cutaneous sensory nerve regeneration.[20,21] Of course, this mechanism remains speculative, because the sensory neural pathways are not well-mapped intranasally. It should be noted that the disordered upper airway breathing of ENS may occur after both radical turbinate excision procedures, partial turbinoplasties, and even mucosal-sparing, submucous resection.[3] For the latter procedure, nerve connections to the mucosa are possibly severed during elevation of a flap between the submucosa and turbinate bone. Although most patients will regenerate these nerves with time, a subset may take a prolonged time to regenerate, or fail to reestablish proper sensory nerve regrowth, leading to loss of sensation.

It has also been posited that patients suffering from ENS may be exacerbated by comorbid mental health disease leading to excessive fixation on nasal symptoms.[22] Many patients after nasal surgery may experience a degree of loss of nasal sensation or emptiness that they do not find overtly concerning, but patients at risk owing to psychiatric factors may inappropriately perseverate in a manner consistent with a form of somatic symptom disorder.[23] This may also be similar to the experience of patients dealing with tinnitus where psychosocial mediators are demonstrated to significantly impact how much tinnitus affects quality of life.[24] Whether these patients could have elements of a preoperative somatic symptom disorder relating to nasal obstruction that leads them to pursue surgery or solely develop this fixation only in the postoperative period owing to maladaptive psychiatric compensatory mechanisms is unknown because adequate longitudinal studies have not been performed. Regardless, practicing clinicians with experience in treating patients with ENS anecdotally report common behavioral tendencies among patients with ENS and even conclude that these features dominate the presentation of ENS. Also, although mental health may be a factor in the degree that a patient suffers with ENS, it should be noted that studies have shown significant improvement of psychiatric comorbidities after appropriate nasally centered ENS treatment.[25–27]

DIAGNOSIS OF EMPTY NOSE SYNDROME

Patients with classic ENS will complain of nasal obstruction that is significantly out of proportion to physical examination, and often include words like "suffocation" or "emptiness" when describing their symptoms. Because the nasal airway appears patent owing to prior turbinate surgery, the symptoms are termed paradoxic, that is, unexpected. In addition, patients with ENS often report dryness of the nose and throat.[3,7] In severe cases, patients become obsessed with nasal airflow and suffocation to the point where they are unable to concentrate or function appropriately in daily life (a phenomenon referred to as aprosexia nasalis).[3,7,10] Because this type of ENS is solely considered to result from postoperative nasal airway changes, virtually all patients with ENS report a history of prior nasal surgery.

In the absence of prior turbinate surgery, other diagnoses must be explored in patients with ENS symptoms; the most commonly considered alternative diagnosis is atrophic rhinitis. In theory, any etiology that destroys nasal tissue can lead to these symptoms. Thus, patients should be asked about inhalational exposure of recreational substances (cocaine, narcotics, etc) or perhaps industrial toxins. Vasculitis (granulomatosis with polyangiitis), IgG4-related disease, and other autoimmune diseases can also cause destruction of turbinate tissue.[28] Minimally invasive endoscopic procedures for sinus and skull base neoplasms will often generate turbinate tissue loss from the surgical approach that ranges from partial to complete removal; the patients may report changes in nasal function, but in general they do not report the same overall morbidity. Interestingly, patients with loss of turbinate tissue owing to inhalational exposures, immune-mediated damage, or tumor surgery rarely describe the full constellation of ENS symptoms.

Traditionally, ENS has been diagnosed based on the clinical history and physical examination; however, the development of the ENS6Q, has provided clinicians a simple tool for ENS diagnosis. The ENS6Q, a recently validated, 6-item questionnaire derived from the 25-item Sinonasal Outcome Test, has demonstrated high sensitivity and specificity for differentiating patients with ENS from those with chronic rhinosinusitis patients and normal controls (**Fig. 2**).[12] A score of 11 out of 30 or greater on the ENS6Q has a specificity of more than 95% and a sensitivity or more than 85% for ENS. The brevity of the ENS6Q, along with its high sensitivity and specificity, make it easily applicable in the clinical setting of otolaryngology.

The cotton test,[3] which also is used for surgical planning, has been validated as a diagnostic or provocative tool to assess patients for ENS (**Fig. 3**).[11] This test involves the application of dry cotton into the site of turbinate tissue loss, typically the inferior meatus. This plug of cotton is intended to replicate the size and shape of each patient's native, preoperative turbinate, and thereby transiently redirect airflow similar to the original turbinate. In many patients suffering from ENS, the beneficial effects of cotton placement can be unexpectedly profound. Despite years of inadequate nasal breathing, a healthy proportion of patients with ENS will experience dramatic improvements in their baseline nasal symptoms (reflected by ENS6Q scoring) within minutes of the cotton test in the office, with a decrease of 7 points from the baseline ENS6Q considered clinically meaningful. It is important that the cotton test is performed without any use of topical decongestants or anesthetics to be reliable.

Recent research has also identified radiologic findings that are highly consistent with ENS. In addition to the markedly decreased inferior turbinate tissue and bone, alternating regions of mucosal thickening along the central septum can be observed on computed tomography scans (**Fig. 4**) with this finding carrying both high specificity and high sensitivity for ENS.[29] It is believed that this striking mounding of the nasal septal mucosa (recently coined the serpentine sign) results from slow, selective hypertrophy (or turbinalization) of the septal mucosal lining over years, as a gradual, compensatory response

Symptom	No Problem/ Not Applicable	Very Mild	Mild	Moderate	Severe	Extremely Severe
Dryness	0	1	2	3	4	5
Sense of diminished nasal airflow (cannot feel air flowing through your nose)	0	1	2	3	4	5
Suffocation	0	1	2	3	4	5
Nose feels too open	0	1	2	3	4	5
Nasal crusting	0	1	2	3	4	5
Nasal burning	0	1	2	3	4	5

Fig. 2. The ENS6Q is a validated questionnaire that can be used to diagnosis ENS and monitor the patient's response to treatment. A score of greater than 11, but especially greater than 15, is suggestive of ENS.

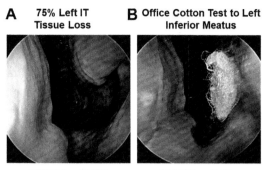

A 75% Left IT
Tissue Loss   **B** Office Cotton Test to Left
Inferior Meatus

ENS6Q = 19/30   ENS6Q = 4/30

Fig. 3. This patient presented with undiagnosed, bilateral (L > R) nasal obstruction and intermittent pain and crusting for more than 6 years. Approximately 75% tissue loss to the left inferior turbinate was seen (*A*), and approximately 60% right inferior turbinate (IT) tissue loss was noted on the right side (not shown). The baseline ENS6Q score was 19 out of 30. No sinus abnormalities were noted on imaging. Without the use of topical sprays, a blinded cotton test was performed in the office, with a dry cotton plug placed into the left inferior meatus fashioned to resemble the anterior head of the IT (*B*). Marked improvement in the patient's subjective nasal breathing (and demeanor) was noted within 2 to 3 minutes, and her ENS6Q score decreased by 15 points to 4 out of 30 (akin to breathing of control subjects). The patient described her breathing as "less effortful and more smooth" with cotton in place, and asked that "whatever was placed in her nose" not be removed. A diagnosis of ENS was confirmed.

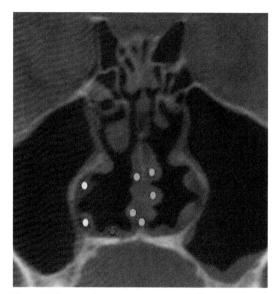

Fig. 4. Progressive development of mounds of mucosal hypertrophy (auto-hypertrophy) often develop in the areas adjacent to sites of inferior turbinate tissue loss in patients with ENS. This computed tomographic (CT) finding has been coined the 'serpentine sign' owing to the alternating dense mounding seen especially along the nasal septum. This patient underwent complete bilateral inferior turbinate (IT) resection more than 25 years before this CT image was taken, and developed peaks or prominent mounds along the nasal septum (*green dots*), nasal floor (*red dot*), and inferior meatus (*yellow dots*) mucosal tissue. The reliability of the serpentine sign for identifying patients with ENS, and the histology of this unusual mucosal tissue, has yet to be established.

of the mucosal lining owing to the decreased turbinate tissue volume.[29,30]

For clinical discussion and surgical planning, ENS may be classified into 3 main subtypes related to degree of tissue resection.[3] Patients with ENS-IT have had inferior turbinate tissue loss, and patients with ENS-MT have experienced middle turbinate partial/complete resections. Patients with resection of both structures are referred to as ENS-both. A fourth classification, ENS-TYPE, is reserved for patients who have a seemingly normal volume of turbinate tissue but still have ENS symptoms such as after conservative submucous resection.

PREVENTION OF EMPTY NOSE SYNDROME

Data measuring the prevalence of ENS after turbinate surgery are limited. Although this may reflect a relatively low incidence, many cases likely go unrecognized or underdiagnosed, and therefore unreported. Another factor that complicates ENS diagnosis and thus prevention is the delay in the development of symptoms over time. Unfortunately, a majority of patients with ENS seem to

report initial satisfaction with their surgical outcome, but then notice a decrease in quality of life owing to the slow onset of ENS symptoms over the subsequent 3 months to more than 5 years after the turbinate-based procedure. Myriad reasons for the latter can be debated, but the subjective nature of each individual's sense of satisfactory nasal breathing, and the gradual onset to notice ENS-like symptoms, have collectively thwarted the ability to make successful links between turbinoplasty surgery and ENS. Patients with ENS are also likely to seek care from a bevy of different surgeons, rather than the original turbinoplasty surgeon, and this pattern precludes the surgeon's development of awareness of this possible association or concern with tissue loss and tissue healing. In fact, surgeons who routinely perform aggressive inferior turbinate resections may believe in the benefit of turbinectomy (because of misperceptions about dissatisfied return patients with complaints), and thus treat all patients in this manner; naturally, these physicians will be less inclined to recognize the signs and symptoms of ENS or interpret turbinate tissue loss as a concern or complication. Importantly, the complaints from patients with ENS are often diffuse and nonspecific and, even under ideal circumstances, a timely and accurate diagnosis can be challenging. The latter highlights the importance of the ENS6Q, because the 6 symptoms queried are commonly shared by ENS sufferers. Moreover, despite these limitations, the correlation between aggressive turbinoplasty surgery (and not other nasal surgeries) with possible development of ENS is striking, and increasing numbers of otolaryngologists support the association of ENS and turbinate tissue loss.[7,9,31]

Because over-resection of inferior turbinate tissue, or poor wound healing after turbinoplasty, seem to be the dominant pathoetiologic factors for ENS, prevention may be achieved via avoidance of aggressive turbinate soft tissue resection. Alternatives to excisional turbinate surgery include submucosal application of limited radiofrequency energy and submucous tissue resection.[32,33] Although each of these tissue-sparing techniques varies, the common goal is the reduction of submucosal tissue bulk and turbinate erectile capacity without violating the turbinate shape or mucosal function of the overlying mucosa and associated nerves and receptors. Evidence has shown that submucous resection can simultaneously improve nasal obstruction while maintaining the functionality of the nasal mucosa such as ciliary beat frequency and mucous transit time.[34] However, despite surface tissue preservation, it is still possible to develop symptoms of ENS, possibly owing to accumulation of tissue loss and tissue contraction at critical airflow sites, exposure of underlying mucosal sites that provide new symptoms, or via destruction of submucosal neurosensory structures. For this reason, it is prudent to consider avoiding routine turbinoplasty except in patients who pass the following assessments: (1) highly symptomatic patients with nasal congestion, (2) moderate-to-severe inferior turbinate tissue hypertrophy clearly obstructing the upper airway and providing symptoms, (3) dynamic changes through the day and night and left-to-right alternating nasal obstruction (implying an inferior turbinate etiology), and (4) nasal congestion symptoms and turbinate hypertrophy that both improve after decongestant application (thus proving that tissue reduction is pleasing to the patient in the office).

It is probably important to assess for any baseline mental health concerns before any planned surgical intervention. The unexpectedly severe comorbid depression and anxiety of patients with ENS is well-documented.[25] As discussed, it is hypothesized that maladaptive neuropsychiatric comorbidities may also be a conduit to the development of ENS.[22,23] Although there are no published data on whether anxiety and/or depression are independent, antecedent, preoperative risk factors for ENS, patients who are fixated on their nasal breathing, and show signs of anxiety about nasal obstruction or nasal packing placement, warrant mindful consideration during surgical planning and patient counseling.

TREATMENT OF EMPTY NOSE SYNDROME

ENS treatment may be classified into medical and surgical treatments. In general, medical treatments are offered to all patients with ENS. If the degree of relief is not sufficient, then surgical treatment (in the office and operating room) can be considered. It should be noted that, even after successful surgical treatment, all patients with ENS should continue medical measures.

Medical Therapy

Medical therapy begins with a focus on moisturization of the nasal lining. Topical moisturization with saline sprays and various emollients may help to relieve the dry sensation, prevent crusting, and decrease pain. Based on physiologic studies of loss of coolness sensation owing to TRPM8,[16] inhaled or applied menthol solutions may benefit patients with ENS through direct stimulation of the available receptors and the perception of nasal cooling.[7,17,18] These repeated treatments may be cumbersome and likely only provide temporary relief without continuous reapplication throughout the day.

In addition to treatment of the physical aspects of ENS, it is important to consider the psychological morbidity of ENS. Patients suffering from a true ENS state have significant, concomitant, documented anxiety and depression[25,27]; both conditions may be unrecognized by the patient, their family, and other treating physicians. It is important to consider a discussion of psychosocial dysfunction with all patients with ENS; this step is especially critical for patients with ENS who are considered for procedural treatments. Consultation with psychiatry or psychology for cognitive–behavioral therapy should be discussed with any patient with a suspected depression and/or anxiety disorder. Surgical intervention for ENS has been shown to improve standardized measurements of anxiety and depression.[25] Even without surgical intervention, there are sporadic but noteworthy reports on the use of targeted mental health therapy alone to address ENS as a somatic symptom disorder,[23] although the severity of ENS symptoms and the degree of turbinate tissue loss was not described.

Because of the common psychiatric comorbidities, physicians treating patients with ENS must screen these patients for depression, anxiety, and somatization disorder as well as other psychiatric conditions. If there is any clinical suspicion of a preclinical psychiatric illness, then a formal psychiatry consult is clearly warranted. Failure to treat the psychiatric comorbidities of ENS will compromise the results of any of the medical and surgical treatments offered to these patients. Obviously, when a psychiatric consultation is made, it is critical for the requesting physician to gain the support and trust of that patient so that follow-through is ensured. Perhaps a reliable way to advance this relationship with a patient with ENS is to validate the patient's observations of altered nasal function and to show comfort with basic awareness of ENS as a clinical entity.

Surgical Therapy

Recently, surgical therapy for ENS has received greater acceptance because evidence of favorable outcomes both in nasal symptom scores and in comorbid mental health domains have been reported.[26,35] In light of the possible neurologic mechanisms of ENS development, it is prudent to allow 6 to 12 months after the inciting surgical event before attempting a corrective procedure. In fact, submucosal filler injections described elsewhere in this article are ideal temporary bulking agents to augment sites of tissue loss, and this procedure can be performed the office. This measure gives time for complete healing of the operated tissues to occur and the regeneration of any neural connections that may resolve the patient's initial complaints.

Young's procedure of temporary nasal closure (either via tissue flaps or with fabricated plugs) has been described as beneficial in atrophic rhinitis.[36,37] Because of the similarity between ENS and acquired atrophic rhinitis, this has also been advocated as potentially beneficial in patients with ENS.[3,7,10] Data on this approach in patients with ENS are sparse.

The majority of surgical treatments for ENS involve reshaping nasal passages to attempt to mimic the previously resected nasal tissue. Simply stated, the goal of the ideal ENS surgery is to restore inferior turbinate bulk to approximate the shape of a normal turbinate; that is, these procedures should be viewed as turbinate reconstruction procedures. Often turbinate reconstruction may not be feasible; in these instances, adding bulk along other nasal surfaces may act to improve the nasal function ascribed to intact inferior turbinate tissue. Planning for surgical intervention should be based on results of the cotton test, which helps to identify sites of deficient turbinate tissue. Surgical correction is directed at filling in these defects (**Fig. 5**). Recreating the shape and position of resected tissues should be considered; however, given the 3-dimensional pattern of turbinate resection, direct replacement of inferior and middle turbinate tissues may not be feasible. Instead, intervention can be targeted toward the nasal floor, lateral nasal wall, or septal tissue with the objective of narrowing the nasal passageways in the area of resection. For example, after middle turbinate resection, where it is not feasible to directly rebuild a neo-turbinate, a submucosal pocket in the adjacent septum with placement of graft material can be considered. Fortunately, reconstructing the inferior turbinate may be

Pre-op   Post-op 4 mo

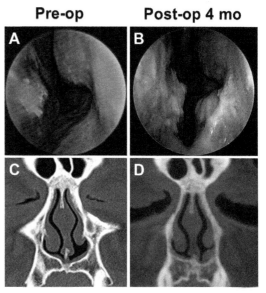

Fig. 5. This patient reported significant left-sided paradoxic nasal obstruction, facial pain and burning sensation with an ENS6Q score of 29 out of 30. Loss of the inferior half of the left inferior turbinate (IT) can be seen both endoscopically (*A*) and radiographically (*C*). Approximately 4 months after inferior meatus augmentation using implanted cadaveric rib, the patient's nasal symptoms had markedly improved, with an ENS6Q score decrease to 5 out of 30. Increased soft tissue volume can be seen in the left inferior meatus (*B*, *D*), leading to altered nasal aerodynamics and resistance.

accomplished at the lateral nasal wall at the level of the inferior meatus.

Numerous materials have been used for submucosal grafting: (1) temporary fillers, (2) acellular dermal allografts, (3) autologous cartilage, and (4) synthetic implants.

Temporary fillers

The submucosal injection of cross-linked hyaluronic acid has been described as a minimally invasive option in patients with ENS.[38] In this report, the commercial product Juvéderm (Allergan, Dublin, Ireland) was used, but a variety of similar products are available; these alternatives are likely to offer similar efficacy. Recent data have also shown efficacy with use of carboxymethyl cellulose gel, originally used for temporary vocal cord augmentation (Prolaryn, Merz, Raleigh, NC).[39] The latter report shows that submucosal filler placement into the inferior meatuses not only significantly improved sinonasal airway complaints (ENS6Q and Sino-nasal Outcome Test-22), but also markedly improved psychiatric (Patient Health Questionnaire-9) and depressive (Generalized Anxiety Disorder-7) symptoms. Interestingly, with slow filler resorption, enrolled patients' rhinologic and nonrhinologic symptoms recrudesced to their baseline severity; this observation supports the notion that nasal airflow and nasal resistance (as regulated by the turbinates), and psychological well-being may be more interdependent than previously appreciated. Submucosal injection of any resorbable gel product is off-label and should be discussed with the patient during the informed consent process. Submucosal instillation of these materials can be accomplished in an office-based setting under local anesthesia. During injection, care must be taken to avoid intravascular injections, which can (theoretically) lead to thromboembolic complications. These materials are absorbed over a time period of 2 to 12 months (and possibly longer). This submucosal transient filler approach can be useful for patients with ENS who are wary of surgery, have severe medical comorbidities that increase the risks of general anesthesia, or have early-onset symptoms after recent turbinoplasty, where tissue healing is still ongoing. The application of submucosal fillers may also serve to hone and/or confirm the results of the office cotton test, by patient affirmation of their satisfaction and blunted ENS symptoms over the weeks and months after gel augmentation in specific nasal sites. Filler placement may also serve as a next step assessment for patients where ENS is suspected, but provocative cotton testing in the office is equivocal for improved breathing. In this setting, having the patient experience their nasal airway function in the presence of a lasting soft tissue filler may help to convince both patient and clinician that indeed soft tissue loss is contributing to ENS-related symptoms. Because of the resorbable nature of said fillers, there is little downside to this approach. In this way, the response to submucosal fillers can serve as a reassuring guide before definitive placement of graft materials with greater bulk and longevity.

Acellular dermis allografts and xenografts

The submucosal implantation of acellular dermis allografts is well described for the surgical treatment of ENS.[3,10,40] Human acellular dermal matrix (such as Alloderm, Allergan, Inc) and porcine submucosal intestine submucosa are designed to integrate into the surrounding soft tissues over time.[41] To place these grafts, submucosal pockets are made under general anesthesia in the target location (typically the lateral wall of the inferior meatus). The graft material can then be rolled tightly and packed into the pocket to narrow the overly patent nasal airway. Multiple sites along the lateral wall of the nasal cavity can be targeted for exogenous graft placement, with implant site guided by sites of obvious tissue loss, cotton test/cotton placement results, and the benefits obtained via submucosal filler placement. Overall data show good efficacy of this approach with lasting benefit,[26] although some users have noted 10% to 30% resorption and breakdown rates for matrix materials. Fragmentation of the submucosal intestine submucosa membrane with the loss of neo-turbinate projection has been reported, making this xenograft less favorable for this application.[41] Patients may have an inflammatory reaction to the allograft, but the acellular nature of this implant makes this reaction exceedingly rare. The use of allografts avoids the time and morbidity associated with autograft harvest. Unfortunately, allograft products are relatively expensive, and are not available in all countries.

Autologous and donor cadaveric cartilage

The biocompatibility, ease of harvest, and decreased materials cost of autologous cartilage makes this an attractive option for ENS surgery. The objectives of cartilage grafting are similar to allograft placement, and the techniques for cartilage placement are analogous to allograft placement techniques. However, cartilage has the advantage of a semirigid consistency, and thus can be shaped and sized to achieve a desired 3-dimensional shape. Autologous cartilage harvested from the ear, nasal septum, or rib can be carved and fashioned to form a cylindrical shape before placing it into a submucosal pocket to simulate the missing turbinate tissue and narrow the nasal airway. Because many patients with ENS will not have adequate septal cartilage owing to previous septoplasty surgery, auricular or costal cartilage may be required, if the surgeon wishes to use an autologous cartilage graft. Submucosal cartilage grafts have been used with success in patients with ENS with good tolerance.[42,43] Like all autologous grafts, graft harvest adds operative time, and the donor site carries its own morbidity. Although not reported to date for ENS, cadaveric rib grafts hold promise for use in ENS turbinate reconstruction. Like cadaveric skin, cadaveric rib is decellularized, irradiated tissue matrix, which should keep rejection and/or rejection rates at low incidence. This hardy material is usually stored at −80°C, and can be thawed and fashioned minutes before use, avoiding the risks and pain for autologous rib harvest. Observational studies on its short- and long-term efficacy are being advanced currently.

Synthetic implants
The use of synthetic implants has been described in ENS reconstructive surgery. These implant options include perforated silicone sheeting or porous polyethylene (MedPor, Stryker Corporation, Kalamazoo, MI).[40,44,45] These materials are nonreactive and designed to allow tissue growth to penetrate the material and improve long term integration. Synthetic implants are relatively inexpensive, and they are easy to obtain in most practices. Because synthetic implants are, by their nature, foreign bodies, extrusion and infection are obvious possible complications. After tissue ingrowth, implant removal owing to scarring is highly challenging if such extraction is warranted.

SUMMARY

The hallmark of ENS is over-resection of turbinate soft issue tissue, or compromised tissue healing, which leads to structural and physiologic changes in the nasal airway. Months to years after a turbinate-related procedure, a minor subset of patients may develop paradoxic symptoms of nasal obstruction and congestion despite the appearance of a patent nasal airway. These patients may also experience nasal burning, crusting, and suffocation—which are felt to be hallmark symptoms associated with ENS. Patients with ENS commonly present with frustration with their symptoms, and with anxiety, depression and somatization disorders layered atop their presenting complaints. Because ENS is an unforeseen complication of surgery, the syndrome is best prevented by avoiding unnecessary and certainly radical turbinate procedures. ENS can now be reliably diagnosed using the ENS6Q questionnaire and tested in the office using the cotton test. Medical treatment of ENS emphasizes nasal moisturization through nasal saline sprays and gels. Patients with severe psychiatric comorbidities should undergo formal psychiatric assessment and treatment as warranted. Surgical therapy for ENS seeks to reestablish turbinate tissue volume (and associated nasal aerodynamics and nasal sensation) through the placement of injectable fillers, allografts, xenografts, cartilage autografts and/or synthetic materials. Although the exact pathoetiologic mechanisms for ENS are not well-understood, symptoms of ENS may be improved through the judicious patient workup, counseling, and application of selected medical and surgical treatments.

REFERENCES

1. Hol MKS, Huizing EH. Treatment of inferior turbinate pathology: a review and critical evaluation of the different techniques. Rhinology 2000;38: 157–66.
2. Moore EJ, Kern EB. Atrophic rhinitis: a review of 242 cases. Am J Rhinol 2001;15:355–61.
3. Chhabra N, Houser SM. The diagnosis and management of empty nose syndrome. Otolaryngol Clin North Am 2009;42:311–30.
4. Hong HR, Jang YJ. Correlation between remnant inferior turbinate volume and symptom severity of empty nose syndrome. Laryngoscope 2016;126: 1290–5.
5. Ophir D, Schindel D, Halperin D, et al. Long-term follow-up of the effectiveness and safety of inferior turbinectomy. Plast Reconstr Surg 1992;90:980–4 [discussion: 985–7].
6. Talmon Y, Samet A, Gilbey P. Total inferior turbinectomy: operative results and technique. Ann Otol Rhinol Laryngol 2000;109:1117–9.
7. Kuan E, Suh J, Wang M. Empty nose syndrome (ENS). J Pharm Sci Res 2015;15:493.
8. Moore GF, Freeman TJ, Ogren FP, et al. Extended follow-up of total inferior turbinate resection for relief of chronic nasal obstruction. Laryngoscope 1985; 95:1095–9.
9. Sozansky J, Houser SM. Pathophysiology of empty nose syndrome. Laryngoscope 2015;125:70–4.
10. Houser SM. Surgical treatment for empty nose syndrome. Arch Otolaryngol Head Neck Surg 2007; 133:858–63.
11. Thamboo A, Velasquez N, Habib ARR, et al. Defining surgical criteria for empty nose syndrome: validation of the office-based cotton test and clinical interpretability of the validated Empty Nose

Syndrome 6-Item Questionnaire. Laryngoscope 2017;127:1746–52.

12. Velasquez N, Thamboo A, Habib ARR, et al. The Empty Nose Syndrome 6-item questionnaire (ENS6Q): a validated 6-item questionnaire as a diagnostic aid for empty nose syndrome patients. Int Forum Allergy Rhinol 2017;7:64–71.

13. Naftali S, Rosenfeld M, Wolf M, et al. The air-conditioning capacity of the human nose. Ann Biomed Eng 2005;33:545–53.

14. Dayal A, Rhee JS, Garcia GJM. Impact of middle vs inferior total turbinectomy on nasal aerodynamics. Otolaryngol Head Neck Surg 2016;155: 518–25.

15. Li C, Farag AA, Leach J, et al. Computational fluid dynamics and trigeminal sensory examinations of empty nose syndrome patients. Laryngoscope 2017;127:176–84.

16. Li C, Farag AA, Maza G, et al. Investigation of the abnormal nasal aerodynamics and trigeminal functions among empty nose syndrome patients. Int Forum Allergy Rhinol 2018;8:444–52.

17. Lindemann J, Tsakiropoulou E, Scheithauer MO, et al. Impact of menthol inhalation on nasal mucosal temperature and nasal patency. Am J Rhinol 2008; 22:402–5.

18. Zhao K, Blacker K, Luo Y, et al. Perceiving nasal patency through mucosal cooling rather than air temperature or nasal resistance. PLoS One 2011;6: e24618.

19. Freund W, Wunderlich AP, Stöcker T, et al. Empty nose syndrome: limbic system activation observed by functional magnetic resonance imaging. Laryngoscope 2011;121:2019–25.

20. Frampton SJ, Pringle M. Cutaneous sensory deficit following post-auricular incision. J Laryngol Otol 2011;125(10):1014–9.

21. Motz KM, Kim YJ. Auriculotemporal syndrome (Frey Syndrome). Otolaryngol Clin North Am 2016;49(2): 501–9.

22. Payne SC. Empty Nose Syndrome: what are we really talking about? Otolaryngol Clin North Am 2009;42:331–7.

23. Lemogne C, Consoli SM, Limosin F, et al. Treating empty nose syndrome as a somatic symptom disorder. Gen Hosp Psychiatry 2015;37:273.e9-10.

24. Andersson G, Westin V. Understanding tinnitus distress: introducing the concepts of moderators and mediators. Int J Audiol 2008;47(Suppl 2): S106–11.

25. Lee TJ, Fu CH, Wu CL, et al. Evaluation of depression and anxiety in empty nose syndrome after surgical treatment. Laryngoscope 2016;126: 1284–9.

26. Leong SC. The clinical efficacy of surgical interventions for empty nose syndrome: a systematic review. Laryngoscope 2015;125:1557–62.

27. Manji J, Nayak JV, Thamboo A. The functional and psychological burden of empty nose syndrome. Int Forum Allergy Rhinol 2018;8:707–12.

28. Hildenbrand T, Weber RK, Brehmer D. Rhinitis sicca, dry nose and atrophic rhinitis: a review of the literature. Eur Arch Otorhinolaryngol 2011;268:17–26.

29. Thamboo A, Velasquez N, Ayoub N, et al. Distinguishing computed tomography findings in patients with empty nose syndrome. Int Forum Allergy Rhinol 2016;6:1075–82.

30. Dholakia SS, Borchard NA, Yan C, et al. The 'serpentine sign': a radiographic screening tool for patients with empty nose syndrome. Paper presented at: American Rhinologic Fall Meeting 2018. Atlanta, GA.

31. Rice DH, Kern EB, Marple BF, et al. The turbinates in nasal and sinus surgery: a consensus statement. Ear Nose Throat J 2003;82:82–4.

32. Chen Y-L, Tan C-T, Huang H-M. Long-term efficacy of microdebrider-assisted inferior turbinoplasty with lateralization for hypertrophic inferior turbinates in patients with perennial allergic rhinitis. Laryngoscope 2008;118:1270–4.

33. Rudes M, Schwan F, Klass F, et al. Turbinate reduction with complete preservation of mucosa and submucosa during rhinoplasty. HNO 2018; 66:111–7.

34. Rhee CS, Kim DY, Won TB, et al. Changes of nasal function after temperature-controlled radiofrequency tissue volume reduction for the turbinate. Laryngoscope 2001;111:153–8.

35. Thamboo A, Dholakia S, Borchard N, et al. Inferior Meatus Augmentation Procedure (IMAP) to treat empty nose syndrome: assessment using validated, disease-specific questionnaires. Otolaryngol Head Neck Surg, in press.

36. el Kholy A, Habib O, Abdel-Monem MH, et al. Septal mucoperichondrial flap for closure of nostril in atrophic rhinitis. Rhinology 1998;36(4):202–3.

37. Lobo CJ, Hartley C, Farrington WT. Closure of the nasal vestibule in atrophic rhinitis–a new non-surgical technique. J Laryngol Otol 1998;112(6): 543–6.

38. Modrzyński M. Hyaluronic acid gel in the treatment of empty nose syndrome. Am J Rhinol Allergy 2011;25:103–6.

39. Borchard N, Dholakia S, Yan C, et al. Use of intranasal submucosal fillers as a transient implant to alter upper airway aerodynamics: implications for the assessment of empty nose syndrome. Int Forum Allergy Rhinol 2019;9(6):681–7.

40. Saafan ME. Acellular dermal (Alloderm) grafts versus silastic sheets implants for management of empty nose syndrome. Eur Arch Otorhinolaryngol 2013;270(2):527–33.

41. Velasquez N, Huang Z, Humphreys IM, et al. Inferior turbinate reconstruction using porcine small

intestine submucosal xenograft demonstrates improved quality of life outcomes in patients with empty nose syndrome. Int Forum Allergy Rhinol 2015;5(11):1077–81.

42. Chang AA, Watson D. Inferior turbinate augmentation with auricular cartilage for the treatment of empty nose syndrome. Ear Nose Throat J 2015; 94(10–11):E14–5.

43. Jung JH, Baguindali MA, Park JT, et al. Costal cartilage is a superior implant material than conchal cartilage in the treatment of empty nose syndrome. Otolaryngol Head Neck Surg 2013; 149(3):500–5.

44. Jiang C, Shi R, Sun Y. Study of inferior turbinate reconstruction with Medpor for the treatment of empty nose syndrome. Laryngoscope 2013;123(5): 1106–11.

45. Tam YY, Lee TJ, Wu CC, et al. Clinical analysis of submucosal Medpor implantation for empty nose syndrome. Rhinology 2014;52(1):35–40.

Correction of Nasal Pinching

Ari J. Hyman, MD[a], Sarah Khayat, MD[b], Dean M. Toriumi, MD[b],*

KEYWORDS

- Revision rhinoplasty • Pinched nasal tip • Complications in rhinoplasty • Alar rim grafts
- Lateral crural strut grafts • Nasal tip contouring • Lateral crural repositioning
- Cephalic malpositioning

KEY POINTS

- The pinched nasal tip can be congenital or iatrogenic.
- The pinched nasal tip deformity characteristically displays a clear demarcation between the tip lobule and the alar lobule, isolating the nasal tip from surrounding nasal subunits.
- Conventional tip modifications, including suturing and cartilage excision or division, which overemphasize narrowing, can weaken support to the alar margin, leading to medial collapse of the alar lobule and tip pinching.
- Methods for correcting the pinched nasal tip require restoration of normal nasal tip architecture and reestablishment of support for the alar margin.
- Techniques that can restore normal tip contour and support to the tip and alar margin include placement of lateral crural strut grafts with or without repositioning and placement of alar rim grafts.

INTRODUCTION

The pinched nasal tip may be congenital owing to inherent weakness, malposition, concave lateral crura, or recurvature of the lateral crus of the lower lateral cartilages. More commonly, however, the pinched tip occurs secondarily as sequelae of prior nasal surgery resulting from an effort to narrow the tip, which deforms the lateral crura and weakens support for the alar margin.[1,2] Rather than a smooth transition from tip lobule to alar lobule on frontal view, the pinched nasal tip is bound by vertical shadows separating the tip and alar lobules, which isolate the tip from its surrounding nasal subunits[2] (**Fig. 1**). On base view, pinching is noted as medial collapse and notching of the alar margin, which disrupts the normal triangular shape seen in a natural-appearing nasal base[2] (**Fig. 2**).

In addition to the cosmetic deficit, loss of support for the alar margin that occurs in the pinched nasal tip deformity can also result in airway compromise.[1] Correcting both the aesthetic and functional deficits typical of the pinched nasal tip deformity requires restoration of tip and alar margin support, which may require structural grafting in the form lateral crural strut grafts with or without repositioning or alar rim grafts. This type of restructuring can be used to restore nasal function and give a natural-appearing nasal tip contour (**Fig. 3**). This article will discuss the anatomic basis for the pinched nasal tip deformity, how to avoid this complication in rhinoplasty, and the advanced techniques employed for its correction.

ANATOMY OF THE ACQUIRED PINCHED NASAL TIP DEFORMITY

Congenital weakness of the lower lateral cartilages, concave lateral crura, and internal recurvature of the lateral crus can predispose or lead to

Disclosure Statement: No disclosures.
[a] Private Practice, Facial Plastic and Reconstructive Surgery, 16311 Ventura Boulevard #600, Encino, CA 91436, USA; [b] Division of Facial Plastic and Reconstructive Surgery, Department of Otolaryngology–Head and Neck Surgery, University of Illinois at Chicago, Chicago, IL 60612, USA
* Corresponding author.
E-mail address: dtoriumi@uic.edu

Facial Plast Surg Clin N Am 27 (2019) 477–489
https://doi.org/10.1016/j.fsc.2019.07.004

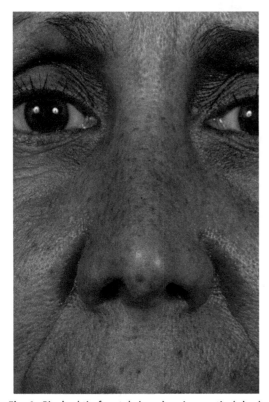

Fig. 1. Pinched tip frontal view showing vertical shadowing between tip and alar lobule.

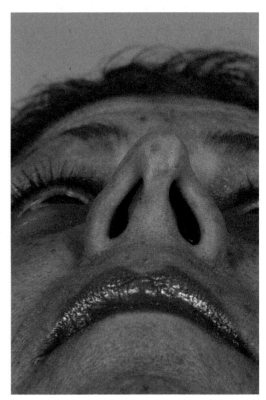

Fig. 2. Pinched tip base view showing medial collapse of the alar margin and peaked nostrils.

primary pinching of the nasal tip. The iatrogenically acquired form is much more common.[1] Many conventionally used tip contouring techniques employ a combination of tip suturing and cartilage excision or division that are designed to narrow the tip and reduce supratip fullness. Many of these techniques can create an unnatural and overly narrow, pinched, and poorly supported tip structure, which appears isolated from the surrounding nasal subunits and detracts from the overall harmony and balance of the nose (**Fig. 4**).

Ideally, the nose should have curvilinear contours and brow tip aesthetic lines that extend from the medial brow to a tip structure that is symmetric and balanced (**Fig. 5**). Favorable tip contour on frontal view is seen as a horizontally oriented highlight with shadowing above in the supratip area and subtly below in the region of the soft tissue facets.[2] The tip highlight extends as an elevated ridge passing in continuity from the tip-defining point to the alar lobule without shadowing demarcating and isolating one from the other. On base view an ideal nasal configuration is triangular in shape with no notching between the tip lobule and the alar lobule (**Fig. 6**). The underlying cartilaginous framework that gives rise to an ideal and natural-appearing nasal tip

contour varies from patient to patient and depends on skin thickness and strength and orientation of the cartilages. Lateral compartment support close to the alar margin is the key structural component. Ideally, the patient would possess caudally positioned lateral crura, in which the caudal margin of the lateral crura lies at close to the same level as the cephalic margin of the lateral crus of lower lateral cartilages (**Fig. 7**). This configuration provides sufficient support for the alar margin and helps counteract retraction. Lateral compartment support can also be provided by placing alar rim grafts or articulated alar rim grafts.

Many of the conventional dome-suturing methods aimed at narrowing the tip decrease the dome angle, medialize, and create an unfavorable relationship between the cephalic and caudal margins of the lateral crura. Cinching the domes together and bringing the caudal margin well below the cephalic margin of the lateral crus lead to pinching of the nasal tip and displacement of alar support, medially weakening support of the alar margin leading to medial displacement, notching, and retraction of the ala. The resultant pinched deformity may not present for many years after surgery as scar contracture ensues. Unfortunately,

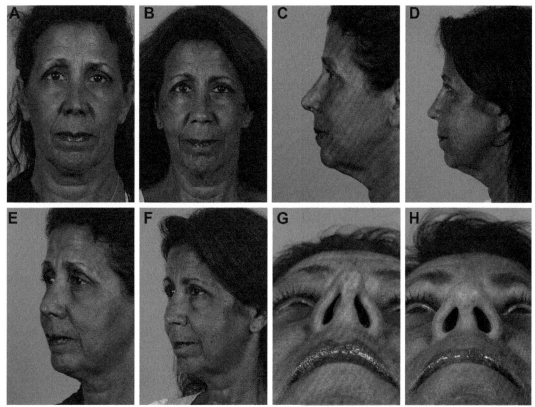

Fig. 3. (*A*) Pinched nasal tip deformity on preoperative frontal view, (*B*) postoperative frontal view, (*C*) Preoperative left lateral view, (*D*) postoperative left lateral view, (*E*) preoperative three-quarters, (*F*) postoperative three-quarters, (*G*) preoperative base view, and (*H*) postoperative base view.

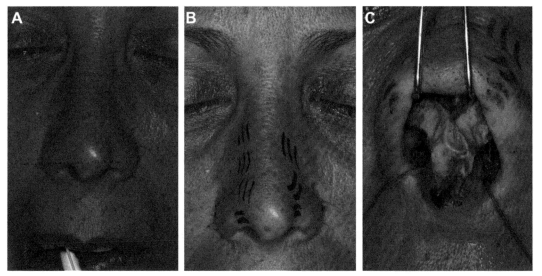

Fig. 4. (*A*) Intraoperative frontal view and (*B*) pinched nasal tip marked to show shadowing before the operation. (*C*) Inspection of the lower lateral cartilages reveals pinching of the tip, concave lateral crura, and cephalic malpositioning.

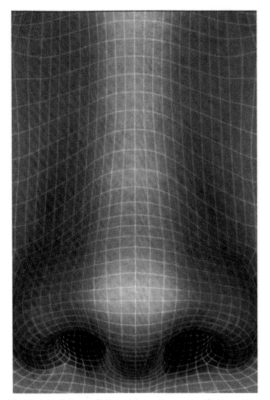

Fig. 5. Ideal frontal view. There is a smooth transition from tip lobule to alar lobule without a line of demarcation. (*From* Toriumi DM, Checcone MA. New concepts in nasal tip contouring. Facial Plast Surg Clin North Am 2009;*17(1):55-90*); with permission.)

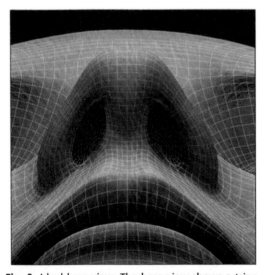

Fig. 6. Ideal base view. The base view shows a triangular shape with no notching between the tip and alar lobule. (*From* Toriumi DM, Checcone MA. New concepts in nasal tip contouring. Facial Plast Surg Clin North Am 2009;*17(1):55-90*); with permission.)

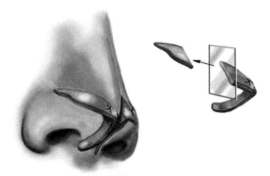

Fig. 7. To provide support to the alar margin, the caudal margin of the lateral crura lies at close to the same level as the cephalic margin of the lateral crura. The inset shows a cross-section of this favorable orientation illustrating how the caudal margin of the lateral crura lies near the same level as the cephalic margin. (*From* Toriumi DM, Checcone MA. New concepts in nasal tip contouring. Facial Plast Surg Clin North Am 2009;*17(1):55-90*); with permission.)

many patients who seek secondary rhinoplasty will present with iatrogenic nasal pinching.

PREOPERATIVE PLANNING AND PREPARATION

The rhinoplasty consultation should begin with a thorough history and focused physical examination. Particular attention is given to the quality and thickness of the nasal skin, which may be compromised from prior surgery. Particularly in the case of revision surgery, ascertaining the patient's perceived cosmetic problem and functional deficits as well as eliciting a chronologic history of all prior nasal surgeries is essential. Although prior operative reports should be reviewed when available, they often may be limited in detail and inconsequential in terms of surgical planning. Additionally, endonasal examination is performed with a rigid endoscope to assess the quality of the nasal lining. The septum may be gently palpated with a cotton tip applicator to assess if remaining septal cartilage is available for use in grafting.

Standardized preoperative photographs should be obtained in all views including frontal, lateral, three-quarter, and base views. Digital image morphing is used in all cases. Imaging improves the surgeon's ability to communicate with patients preoperatively regarding possible changes to be made to the nose, and this in turn helps the surgeon better understand the patient's aesthetic preferences. Imaging may help prevent a dissatisfied patient should the surgeon and the patient's aesthetic goals be misaligned.[3] Close attention is given to any existing asymmetries in alar insertion height, alar retraction, or notching. If repositioning is planned, potential for nostril asymmetry postoperatively is discussed with the patient.[4] The surgeon should also discuss that structural grafting may be required and that harvest of costal or auricular cartilage may be necessary if adequate septal cartilage is not available. The increased stiffness of the nose that occurs as a result of structural grafting postoperatively should also be discussed.

OPERATIVE TECHNIQUE

Understanding the correlation between the external nasal contour and the shape of the underlying tip structures and how this contributes or detracts from the creation of a pinched nasal tip with poor alar support is imperative if correcting this deformity is to be successful. Techniques designed to restore support to the alar margin (lateral compartment) and give strength to and reestablish a favorable tilt of the lateral crus such that the caudal margin lies in close to the same plane as the cephalic margin will help to restore a more natural-appearing and ideal nasal tip contour and correct nasal tip pinching. These techniques include lateral crural strut grafts with or without repositioning and in some cases placement of alar rim grafts.[3]

OPENING THE NOSE

Rhinoplasty can be approached endonasally; however, it is the opinion of the senior author (DMT) that the open approach offers enhanced exposure and is preferred when correcting the iatrogenic pinched nasal tip requiring placement of lateral crural strut grafts with repositioning. The surgeon begins by injecting 1% lidocaine with 1:100,000 epinephrine into the septum, along the marginal incisions, over the nasal dorsum and middle vault and in the nasal tip area. Injection of the septum helps to assist in hydrodissecting the mucoperichondrial flaps off of the septum and helps gauge how much remaining cartilaginous septum may be available for use in reconstruction. At least 10 minutes should pass before the procedure is initiated to allow the full vasoconstrictive effect to set in. If the patient is presenting for a revision rhinoplasty, he or she will likely require auricular or costal cartilage harvest for grafting. Irrespectively, it is often advantageous to first open the nose prior to harvesting cartilage grafts to determine the status of the existing septum and better understand the specific cartilage needs necessary for reconstruction.

A midcolumellar inverted-V incision is made in the columella using a #11 scalpel. If the prior surgeon did not use an external approach, depending on the planned final projection of the tip, the columellar incision can either be positioned closer to the tip if significant deprojection is planned or closer to the lip should significant projection be planned. However, in most revision cases, the incision will be dictated by the location of the midcolumellar scar; it is the authors' practice to make an incision just above the prior scar with the intention of excising the scar with a #11 blade prior to closure, assuming the wound can be closed without significant tension after excision (**Fig. 8**). Bilateral marginal incisions are then made using a #15 scalpel; these incisions are connected to the marginal extensions of the columellar incision. Sharp dissection, rather than blunt dissection with spreading, is performed using converse scissors to elevate the skin envelope. Sharp dissection helps to ensure maintenance of the subdermal plexus and decreases postoperative swelling and edema. Three-point retraction with the assistance of a secondary surgeon helps to ensure dissection remains in the correct surgical plane. A Joseph periosteal elevator is used to elevate the periosteum off the bony dorsum remaining in a narrow pocket.

Any reconstruction of the bony pyramid in the form of rasping or osteotomies should be undertaken prior to harvesting septal cartilage for grafting. This will help avoid destabilizing the keystone area. After completing the upper one-third reconstruction, a septoplasty can then be performed either through a separate Killian incision or by dissection between the medial crura, maintaining a 1.5 cm L-strut both dorsally and caudally. Of note, a backcut is often made at the superior

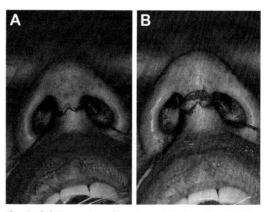

Fig. 8. (A) Base view showing midcolumellar incision marked prior to excision of scar and (B) excised columellar scar.

aspect of the septum as to maintain a larger component of cartilage at the keystone attached to the ethmoid. The midvault is next addressed, and the upper two-thirds are contoured based on anticipated final tip position prior to addressing the lower one-third of the nose.

STABILIZING THE BASE

Prior to reconstruction of the nasal tip with repositioning or grafting of the lateral crura, it is essential to first ensure stability of the nasal base. Close attention is given to first ensuring a stable and midline L-strut has been established as this creates the foundation for nasal tip reconstruction. Careful assessment of preoperative photographs can help identify inherent facial asymmetries as well as any deviation of the posterior or anterior septal angle with tilting of the columella, deviation of the nasal tip, the dorsum, lip or dentition with respect to the midline glabella. Facial asymmetries should be discussed with the patient preoperatively, and any tilt or deviations must be corrected prior to stabilizing the nasal base to avoid persistence of deviation of the nasal tip postoperatively. Once the midline has been established, attention can then be turned toward stabilizing the nasal base onto either an excessive caudal septum, a caudal septal extension graft, or in some instances a caudal septal replacement graft. Caudal septal extension grafts are secured end-to-end with the caudal septum with bilateral extended spreader grafts and stabilized further with slivers of cartilage or ethmoid bone to splint the graft to the existing caudal septum (**Fig. 9**). In patients found to have a severely deviated caudal portion of the L-strut, a caudal septal replacement graft with a subtotal septal reconstruction should be strongly considered. Although more complex, a subtotal septal reconstruction traditionally requires less cartilage than securing a caudal septal extension graft to a severely deviated caudal septum.[5] It is worth noting that the caudal septal extension graft is the only completely straight graft used in the nose, and for this reason, septal cartilage is preferentially used so as to mitigate the risk of warping or future deformity. Any deviation in this graft will translate into deviation of the nasal tip.

The next step in stabilizing the nasal base before further tip contour work is performed is to preliminarily secure the medial crura to the septum or septal extension graft with a 4-0 plain gut suture on an SC-1 needle. Tip rotation, ala-columellar relationship, projection, length, and degree of columellar show are assessed at this point. If the surgeon is pleased with this position, a follow-up 5-0 PDS suture is placed to further secure the

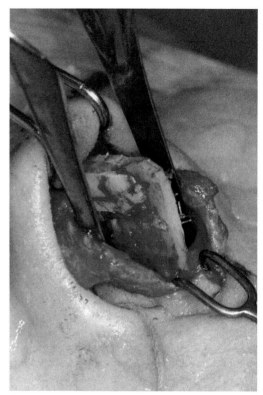

Fig. 9. A caudal septal extension graft is secured end-to-end with the caudal septum, with bilateral extended spreader grafts and stabilized further with perforated ethmoid bone to splint the graft to the existing caudal septum.

medial and intermediate crura to the caudal septum (**Fig. 10**). Pulling the medial crura and columella anteriorly prior to placement of these sutures will open the nasolabial angle, increase projection, and shorten the upper lip, whereas setting the medial crura back toward the posterior septal angle will create a more acute nasolabial angle, deproject the nose, and lengthen the lip (**Fig. 11**). Care must be taken in applying these sutures, as asymmetries can affect tip position or tip symmetry.

GRAFTING MATERIAL

In most revision rhinoplasty operations, there is inadequate septal cartilage available for the structural grafting required to restore a natural tip contour and adequate alar margin support. Auricular cartilage can be harvested but is softer, weaker, and thicker than grafts fashioned from costal cartilage and usually not adequate in length for bilateral lateral crural strut grafts.[6] If auricular cartilage is harvested, a posterior conchal incision is used to minimize the chance of ear deformity or change

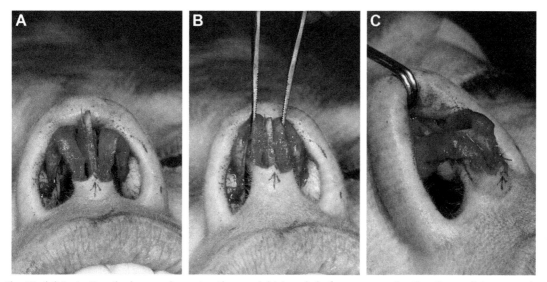

Fig. 10. (*A*) Projecting the base and opening the nasolabial angle before reapproximating the medial crura to the caudal septum (*B*) and after (*C*) from 2 angles.

in position (**Fig. 12**). A bolster is sewn in place for 14 days postoperatively.

Costal cartilage is the authors' preferred grafting source in cases requiring lateral crural strut grafts. Costal cartilage can be harvested from an 11 mm incision (**Fig. 13**), particularly when the seventh rib is used. A larger incision may be employed if the surgeon is less experienced or if an inframammary incision is made within a natural skin crease in the case of sixth rib harvest. The authors prefer to use the seventh rib for several reasons. One, the cartilaginous seventh rib tends to be straighter and

longer. Additionally, the sixth rib often contains a genu that will shorten the straight segment available for grafting. Furthermore, the seventh rib tends to sit below the diaphragm and therefore poses less risk of injury to the pleura.[7] One drawback of its use is the need to place the incision outside of the natural inframammary skin crease, and this necessitates the use of a smaller incision. Costal perichondrium is often harvested from the superior aspect of the ribs, which can be used to camouflage grafts or smooth an irregular dorsum. In some cases, the costal perichondrium is

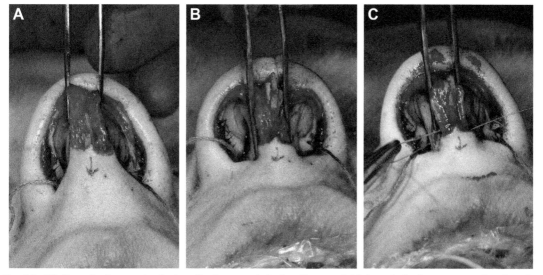

Fig. 11. (*A*) Deprojecting and suturing the base and closing the nasolabial angle before reapproximating the medial crura to the caudal septum (*B*) and after (*C*) from 2 angles.

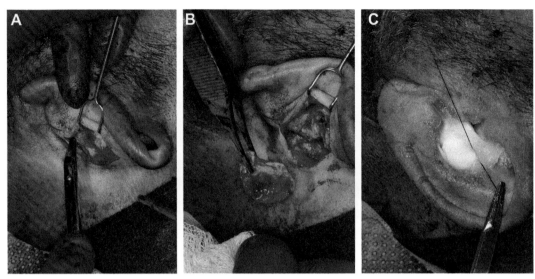

Fig. 12. (*A*) Auricular cartilage harvest through a posterior conchal incision. (*B*) The harvested cartilage is shown, (*C*) followed by bolster placement.

maintained attached to the superior surface of the rib and maintained on the graft, which adds a protective surface that can be placed facing the vestibular mucosa in the case of lateral crural strut grafts.

LATERAL CRURAL STRUT GRAFTS/ REPOSITIONING

Once the base has been stabilized onto a midline L-strut, the next task is to determine which tip reconstructive maneuvers are required to alter tip contour in a way that alleviates pinching and creates a natural-appearing nasal tip structure. One such powerful technique that can accomplish this is placement of lateral crural strut grafts with or without repositioning. Lateral crural strut grafts

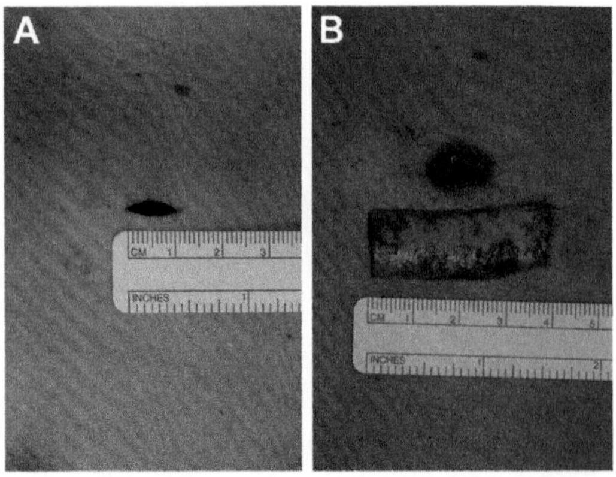

Fig. 13. Rib cartilage harvest. (*A*) An 11 mm incision (*B*) is made overlying the seventh rib, and sufficient costal cartilage is harvested for grafting.

can flatten round or overly convex crura, give support to the alar margin, correct external valve collapse, efface the demarcation of tip and alar lobules, and restore support to weakened or damaged lateral crura.[4] Placement of lateral crural strut grafts requires that the vestibular mucosa be dissected from the undersurface of the native lateral crura. This dissection is facilitated by first hydrodissecting with 1% lidocaine with 1:100,000 epinephrine, with the bevel of the needle flat against the undersurface of the cartilage (**Fig. 14**).[3]

Blunt dissection is easily performed with a Converse scissor starting at the caudal margin, with dissection progressing laterally toward the sesamoid cartilages once the plane is established. Additionally, dissection is carried medial to the natural dome. Completely freeing the lateral crura allows for unhindered domal repositioning if desired. Moving the dome laterally will increase projection similar to lateral crural steal. Moving the dome medially will deproject the tip, similar to a medial crural steal. However, unlike the classic crural steal maneuvers, by first stabilizing the nasal base and then freeing the lateral crus completely, other variables related to the nose such as rotation and length are independent of this change in dome position. Tip projection or deprojection is thus limited only by the length of available medial or lateral crura or by limitations in the skin envelope.

Once the lateral crus of the lower lateral cartilages is free, the surgeon can determine if repositioning is to be performed, and if so, what position would be ideal. If no repositioning is performed, a

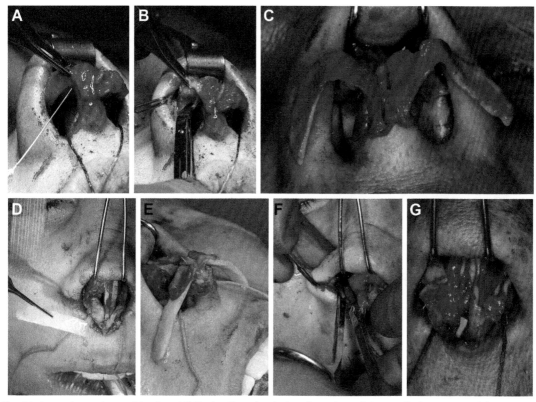

Fig. 14. Lateral crural repositioning. (*A*) Hydrodissection helps dissection of the vestibular mucosa. (*B*) Dissection is performed toward the sesamoid cartilages and medially to the dome. (*C*) The lateral crura are completely freed. (*D*) Lateral crural strut grafts showing a 45° bevel toward the dome. (*E*) The lateral crural strut grafts in place with a slight concavity facing the airway. (*F*) A pocket is created at the lateral end of the marginal incision. (*G*) The tip structure with the grafts placed into pockets.

pocket is made extending at the angle of the lateral crus. This pocket will house the lateral extent of the graft. These cartilage grafts typically measure between 28 to 32 mm in length, 4 to 5 mm in height, and 1 to 2 mm in thickness. The medial edge of the graft is beveled at a 45° angle and positioned just short of the dome, with the cephalic margin close but not beyond the cephalic edge of the native lateral crus. The apex of the angled end of the lateral crural strut graft is placed along the caudal margin of the lateral crura close to but not into the dome. This angulation will facilitate the elevation of the caudal margin of the lateral crura to create a favorable orientation or tilt to the lateral crus. The authors routinely carve these grafts early in the operation to allow time for grafts to display their natural tendency to warp.

Lateral crural strut grafts should ideally be placed with a concave surface facing the airway. If a convex surface faces into the nose it may impinge on the airway. Grafts are sutured to the undersurface of the lateral crus with the knot placed on the superior surface away from the vestibular skin to avoid extrusion. This maneuver will flatten overly convex lateral crura. This is followed with a dome suture to further flatten the domes and create a favorable orientation along the long axis of the cartilage.[8] This suture causes an upward tilt of the caudal margin and a downward tilt of the cephalic margin, helping to restore support to the alar margin, decreasing supratip volume and helping to create a defined horizontal ridge between the tip lobule and alar lobule obliterating the pinched tip, where an unnatural vertical shadow disrupts the transition from tip to the ala. The dome suture is oriented such that it is angled closer to the caudal margin medially and directed toward the cephalic margin laterally. An interdomal suture is then placed to bring the 2 domes into appropriate approximation and secure the dome structure to the anterior projection of the caudal septal extension graft.

The decision whether to reorient depends on the angle formed by the horizontal axis of the lateral crus and the dorsal septum. Ideally, the

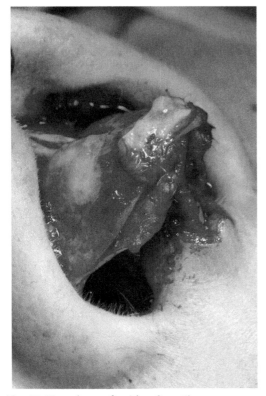

Fig. 15. Tip onlay graft with soft cartilage.

angle should be greater than 30°. If this number is less than 30° to 35°, the authors routinely reposition. In a retrospective chart review of 100 consecutive primary rhinoplasty patients and 100 consecutive secondary rhinoplasty patients, Constantian found that most of the patients seeking both primary and secondary rhinoplasty were identified as having either ball or boxy tips and were noted to have malpositioned lateral crura (74% and 72%, respectively).[9] In fact, most patients in the study (68% of primary rhinoplasty patients and 87% of secondary rhinoplasty patients) had malpositioned lateral crura defined as lateral crura pointing toward the ipsilateral medial canthus versus the lateral canthus. Of note, lengthening the caudal septum by way of caudal septal extension, which is often necessary in revision surgery, will accentuate cephalic malposition by making the angle between the septum and lateral crura more acute. If the lateral crura, in the face of septal lengthening, are not also repositioned caudally, it is possible that the nose will appear unnatural with exacerbation of the cephalic malposition. In contradistinction to lengthening the septum, if the nose is to be shortened, the acute angle between the lateral crura and the midline septum will increase, creating a more favorable orientation.[10]

The next task is placement of the lateral end of the lateral crural strut graft in a newly created

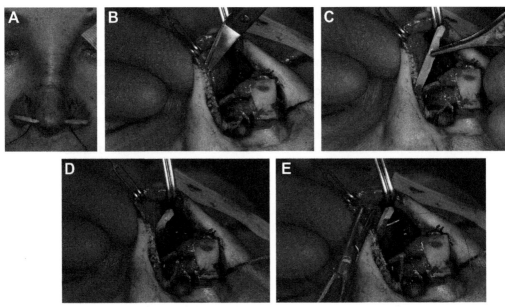

Fig. 16. (*A*) Alar rim grafts. Alar rim grafts typically measure 12 to 15 mm in length. (*B*) Sharp dissection of the premarginal skin is performed to make a narrow pocket. (*C, D*) The rim graft is placed into the pocket. (*E*) A suture is passed through soft tissue and around the graft for stabilization. The medial end of the graft can be bruised with a Brown Adson forceps to help prevent visibility of the graft.

pocket that extends toward the pyriform aperture. This pocket should be long enough for the graft to sit without bowing. Pocket creation begins at the lateral end of the marginal incision with dissection progressing just within or inferior to the supra-alar groove. Placement of the graft into a pocket superior to the supra-alar groove can lead to undesirable fullness and compromise the aesthetic result. Dissecting in a more caudal direction toward the lip is performed in cases of retracted nostrils or to lower a high alar base insertion. After placement of the lateral crural strut grafts is complete, the skin envelope is returned, and lateral and frontal views are observed. If further tip or infratip lobular augmentation is needed, a horizontally oriented tip onlay graft made from soft cartilage can be sutured across the domes with a 6-0 Monocryl suture. Although any appropriately camouflaged piece of cartilage will suffice for this purpose, the authors prefer the use a soft piece of cartilage obtained from the most lateral aspect of the lateral crus (**Fig. 15**).[3] Tip or infratip onlay grafts can be positioned more cranially or caudally with varying widths and thicknesses to further manipulate projection, tip width, and refinement and alter the degree of supratip and infratip break.

RIM GRAFT

If lateral crural strut graft placement with or without repositioning and dome-refining techniques cannot fully restore a smooth transition from tip

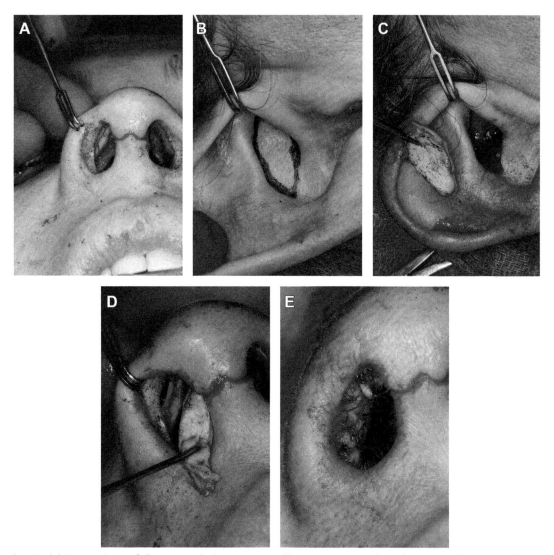

Fig. 17. (*A*) Composite graft harvest and placement. Insufficient mucosa to close the marginal incision is shown. (*B*) Cymba concha is marked prior to harvest. (*C*) Composite graft is harvested. (*D*) Composite graft placed prior to suturing. (*E*) Composite graft sutured in position.

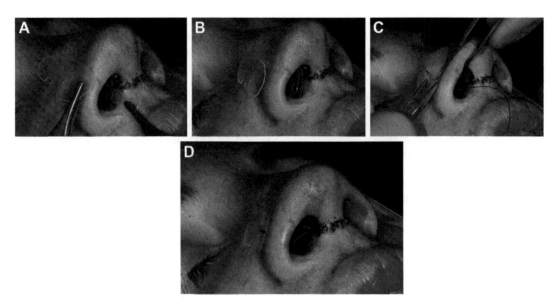

Fig. 18. (*A*) Sidewall splint placement. Fluoroplastic septal splints are cut to appropriate size (*B*) and placed along the vestibular mucosa and over the opposing ala (*C*). The splint is secured with 3-0 nylon suture. (*D*) Following closure.

to alar lobule, the surgeon may resort to using alar rim grafts to salvage the ideal tip contour. These grafts can be placed by creating a narrow pocket just caudal to the marginal incision.[11] These grafts often measure 2 to 3 mm in width and 12 to 15 mm in length (**Fig. 16**). Alar rim grafts help to lower the alar margin and create a more favorable triangular shape on base view.[1] Additionally rim grafts can help provide a smooth transition between the nasal tip and alar lobule, which is useful in treating the pinched nasal tip. The medial margin of the graft is often bruised with a brown Adson forceps to reduce visibility, and a 6-0 Monocryl suture is placed around the medial end of the graft for fixation.

CLOSURE

A single midline subcutaneous 6-0 Monocryl suture is placed in most instances to align the transcolumellar incision and decrease any wound tension. Interrupted 7-0 nylon vertical mattress sutures are placed in the midline and the 2 lateral apices of the inverted V to slightly evert the wound edges. A 6-0 fast-absorbing plain gut is used to close the remainder of the incision. The marginal incisions are closed with 5-0 chromic gut suture in an interrupted fashion. If the vestibular skin has been dissected as in the case of placement of lateral crural strut grafts, a minimum of 2 sutures should be placed. If there is inadequate vestibular lining, closure of the marginal incision will lead to notching. In these cases, composite grafts from

the concha cymba are used (**Fig. 17**).[12] The septum is closed in a quilting fashion using a 4-0 plain gut suture. In all cases of lateral crural strut graft placement with repositioning, lateral wall splints are used (Fluoroplastic septal splints, Medtronic Xomed, Jacksonville, Florida) (**Fig. 18**).[3] Finally, the nose is taped, and a cast is applied. Antibiotic ointment should be applied to all incisions.

ADDITIONAL CONSIDERATIONS

In addition to the commonly quoted complications possible with any rhinoplasty operation including bleeding, scarring, infection, and aesthetic or functional deficits, unique to the use of lateral crural strut grafting is the risk of increased stiffness of the nose owing to the use of cartilage grafting and suspension of the nasal tip onto a rigid caudal septal extension graft. Additionally, the use of these grafts can increase base width and flare of the nostril, so the need for alar base surgery is increased when this maneuver is utilized. Nostril asymmetry is a potential complication if not properly executed. However, this technique is a useful means by which to correct preoperative nostril asymmetries when they exist.

SUMMARY

The pinched nasal tip deformity may be congenital but more often results secondarily as a sequela of prior nasal surgery. Conventional tip surgery techniques including suturing and cartilage excision, which overemphasizes tip narrowing, often deform the lateral crura and weaken support for the alar margin. The pinched nasal tip is characterized by the demarcation between the nasal tip and the alar lobule isolating the tip from the surrounding nasal subunits. Lateral crural strut grafts with or without repositioning offer the surgeon a powerful maneuver that can help correct this functional and aesthetic deformity and restore a natural appearance to the nasal tip.

REFERENCES

1. Paun S, Trenite G. [Chapter: 19]. Correction of the pinched nasaltip deformity. In: Babak A, Murphy MR, William N, editors. Master techniques in rhinoplasty. Saunders; 2011. p. 235–44.
2. Toriumi DM, Checcone MA. New concepts in nasal tip contouring. Facial Plast Surg Clin North Am 2009;17(1):55–90, vi.
3. Toriumi DM, Asher SA. Lateral crural repositioning for treatment of cephalic malposition. Facial Plast Surg Clin North Am 2015;23(1):55–71.
4. Gunter JP, Friedman RM. lateral crural strut graft: technique and clinical applications in rhinoplasty. Plast Reconstr Surg 1997;99(4):943–52.
5. Toriumi DM. Subtotal septal reconstruction: an update. Facial Plast Surg 2013;29(6):492–501.
6. Kim DW, Ali MJ. Complications in head and neck surgery. Second edition 2009. p. 559–76.
7. Jung D-H, Choi S-H, Moon H-J, et al. A cadaveric analysis of the ideal costal cartilage graft for Asian rhinoplasty. Plast Reconstr Surg 2004;114(2):545–50.
8. Toriumi DM. New concepts in nasal tip contouring. Arch Facial Plast Surg 2006;8(3):156–85.
9. Constantian MB. The boxy nasal tip, the ball tip, and alar cartilage malposition: variations on a theme–a study in 200 consecutive primary and secondary rhinoplasty patients. Plast Reconstr Surg 2005;116(1):268–81.
10. Toriumi DM, Bared A. Revision of the surgically overshortened nose. Facial Plast Surg 2012;28(4):407–16.
11. Rohrich RJ, Raniere J, Ha RY. The alar contour graft: correction and prevention of alar rim deformities in rhinoplasty. Plast Reconstr Surg 2002;109(7):2495–505.
12. Losquadro WD, Bared A, Toriumi DM. Correction of the retracted alar base. Facial Plast Surg 2012;28(2):218–24.

Postsurgical Alar Retraction
Etiology and Treatment

Wee Tin K. Kao, MD[a], Richard E. Davis, MD[b,c],*

KEYWORDS

- Rhinoplasty • Post-rhinoplasty complications • Post-surgical alar retraction • Pinched tip
- Alar notching • Articulated alar rim graft

KEY POINTS

- Post-surgical alar retraction (PSAR) is a common complication following overresection of the lateral crus with the cephalic trim technique.
- Upward (cephalic) displacement of the weakened lateral crural remnant occurs when the skeletal void shrinks from progressive epithelial contracture.
- The external approach is used for correction of PSAR.
- PSAR treatment requires release of the entrapped crural-rim complex followed by 3-fold stabilization of the tip complex with septal extension graft placement, lateral crural tensioning, and articulated alar rim graft placement.

INTRODUCTION

Surgical refinement of the unsightly nasal tip remains one of the most difficult procedures in aesthetic surgery. Successful tip refinement requires altering the complex and fragile three-dimensional skeletal architecture to achieve an attractive and natural tip contour, all while maintaining adequate nasal airflow and long-term structural stability. The process is made even more difficult by the powerful and potentially harmful forces of wound-healing that can distort and deform a weakened tip complex and thereby ruin the surgical outcome. The challenge of creating a sturdy skeletal framework that can withstand the chronic and insidious forces of wound healing, while simultaneously achieving exacting changes in tip size, shape, and/or positioning, is indeed formidable, and failure to achieve stable long-term tip support is one of the most common causes of rhinoplasty treatment failure. Instability of the tip complex is most often rooted in overaggressive skeletal excision, which is frequently compounded by a failure to properly reconstitute interconnections of the surgically modified skeletal framework. Moreover, these fundamental errors are amplified by chronic soft tissue contracture that progressively distorts the shape, position, and/or symmetry of the surgically weakened tip complex. Because distortion of a surgically destabilized tip may also be exacerbated by aging, disease, and/or mimetic movement, the adverse effects of skeletal destabilization may worsen for decades in the susceptible nose.

Among the most conspicuous tip deformities commonly resulting from skeletal overresection, retraction of the alar rim is arguably one of the most objectionable because it results in a stigmatic and unsightly tip complex with misshapen and

Disclosures: None.
[a] Division of Facial Plastic and Reconstructive Surgery, Department of Otolaryngology, University of Miami Miller School of Medicine, 1120 Northwest 14th Street, 5th Floor, Miami, FL 33136, USA; [b] Facial Plastic and Reconstructive Surgery Fellowship, The University of Miami Miller School of Medicine, Miami, FL, USA; [c] The Center for Facial Restoration, 1951 Southwest 172nd Avenue, Suite 205, Miramar, FL 33029, USA
* Corresponding author. The Center for Facial Restoration, 1951 Southwest 172nd Avenue, Suite 205, Miramar, FL 33029.
E-mail address: DrD@davisrhinoplasty.com

overly prominent nostril openings. Triggered by overresection of the cephalic margin of the lateral crus (the so-called "cephalic trim" technique), which preserves a "rim strip" of varying width (**Fig. 1**B), and then intensified by the chronic forces of contracture acting on the surgically weakened crural remnant (**Fig. 1**C), postsurgical alar retraction (PSAR) is highly resistant to effective treatment. In this article we describe using the external rhinoplasty approach to correct PSAR by: (1) lysing adhesions to release and reposition the retracted crural remnant and the attached alar rim (**Fig. 1**D), what we have termed the "crural-rim complex"; (2) strengthening and stabilizing the L-strut and central tip compartment using a septal extension graft (SEG) (**Fig. 1**E); (3) using the lateral crural tensioning (LCT) technique to re-engineer tip dynamics so as to stabilize the newly repositioned crural remnant and simultaneously generate

tensioning forces that restore intrinsic sidewall support and tip contour (**Fig. 1**F); and (4) fortifying alar rim stability by providing direct skeletal support with articulated alar rim grafts (AARG) that are integrated into the tip framework (**Fig. 1**G). By using this stepwise structural treatment paradigm, we have successfully corrected, or greatly improved, severe PSAR in the preponderance of revision rhinoplasty cases.

NASAL TIP SUPPORT

It is important to begin any discussion of PSAR with a review of nasal tip support. In the naturally healthy and attractive nose, strong soft tissue interconnections and a stable skeletal framework combine to form a sturdy and resilient tip complex that can withstand the test of time and maintain shape constancy. However, to surgically alter the

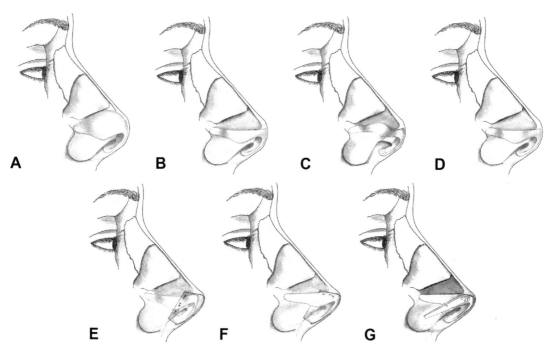

Fig. 1. Schematic illustration of postsurgical alar retraction treatment protocol. (*A*) Congenital bulbous cupping with dome-like convexity of the lateral crus. (*B*) Overresection of the cephalic border of the lateral crus using the "cephalic trim" technique. Note the large skeletal void and the narrow crural remnant (ie, the rim strip). (*C*) Deformation of the surgically weakened lateral crural remnant secondary to cicatricial contracture of the denuded vestibular epithelium. Note cephalic retraction of the crural-rim complex and concomitant concave collapse of the weakened crus. (*D*) Adhesion release and mobilization of the crural-rim complex with initial restoration of normal alar rim contour. (*E*) Septal extension graft placement for optimization of tip contour and to counteract forces generated by crural tensioning. Note modest increase in tip projection and nasal length to improve profile aesthetics. (*F*) Resuspension of the crural remnant from the tip-defining point to stretch and "tension" the tip framework for favorable tip dynamics. Note crural length reduction (using lateral crural steal) to eliminate redundant crural length and precisely match the newly modified sidewall span. (*G*) Placement of a cantilevered articulated alar rim graft to provide direct stationary skeletal support to the repositioned crural-rim complex. Note bridging of the tip and alar lobules by articulated alar rim graft placement thereby restoring strength and optimal shape to the alar ridge.

size, shape, or position of the tip complex using the external rhinoplasty approach, degloving the tip framework by necessity eliminates or weakens many of the secondary support mechanisms that ensure tip stability. Unless a sturdy and durable skeletal framework is reconstituted to prevent future changes in tip shape, a satisfactory long-term result is highly improbable. The large number of patients seeking secondary rhinoplasty to correct delayed tip deformities resulting from skeletal destabilization are testament to the paramount importance of long-term structural stability.

PRIMARY NASAL TIP SUPPORT: ALAR CARTILAGES

Primary structural support of the healthy and attractive tip complex is derived from the paired lower lateral cartilages (LLC). The size, shape, and positioning of the LLC vary widely, even among attractive noses, but mirror-image symmetry of the LLC is a near universal attribute of the attractive nasal tip. In addition to governing nasal tip shape, the conjoined LLC also govern the size, shape, and dynamics of the anterior nasal airway. Hence, the LLC perform a dual role as aesthetic and functional entities, and surgical alterations in tip architecture can enhance or impede airway function. There are also wide variations in the natural strength of the LLC among individuals, ranging from rigid and firm, to weak and flimsy. In the overly wide, bulbous, or boxy nasal tip complex, exceedingly weak LLC are surprisingly common. Furthermore, in noses with naturally weak LLC, unsightly tip morphologies, such as ptosis, splaying, or inadequate projection, are also common; and patients who seek tip refinement for these deformities are often at increased risk for adverse outcomes because of the pathologic weakness of their LLC. On a microscopic level, the LLC are biomechanically weaker (relative to septal cartilage) with less densely packed collagen fibers when viewed under high-resolution electron microscopy.[1] The lateral crura also measure only 0.7 mm in thickness,[2,3] which contributes to the typically delicate nature of the tip complex, and which makes reliable reconstruction using donor cartilage of comparable thickness virtually impossible.

The three-dimensional shape of the LLC not only influences tip morphology, it can also contribute to the architectural strength and stability of the nasal tip complex. In the bulbous nasal tip, cupping of the LLC produces a dome-like convexity of the lateral crura that confers additional shape-derived strength to the lower nasal sidewall (**Fig. 1**A). Although the cartilage itself may be thin and pathologically weak, cupping serves to compensate for the intrinsic weakness of the lateral crura by providing shape-derived stability.[4] The architectural stability of a dome is well recognized. As a series of infinite interlocking arches with no angles or corners, a dome distributes weight evenly in all directions so that no component is subjected to a disproportionate structural load. Dome-shaped buildings have withstood hurricanes, EF4 level tornadoes, and earthquakes[5,6] with no significant damage, and one of the only structures left quasi-intact after the first nuclear bomb attack on Hiroshima, Japan, was the Genbaku dome atop the capitol building.[7] Not surprisingly, anatomic cupping of bulbous lateral crura also imparts dome-like architectural stability to otherwise anatomically weak lateral crura. However, because bulbous cupping is also highly conspicuous and cosmetically objectionable, bulbosity is a common underlying motivation for tip rhinoplasty. Traditionally, refinement of the bulbous tip has been predicated on aggressive "trimming" of the lateral crura (see **Fig. 1**B), but the disagreeable cosmetic appearance of the bulbous nose frequently prompts crural overresection.[4,8–11] The excessive loss of crural volume, coupled with the concomitant loss of dome-like structural stability, then combine to severely destabilize the lateral crura and trigger progressive tip deformation, an all too common occurrence in tip rhinoplasty (see **Fig. 1**C).

Moreover, structural instability generated by the cephalic trim technique is compounded by loss of the nasal scroll, the interlocking junction of the upper and LLC that reinforces the lower nasal sidewall. Following overresection of the bulbous tip, the once stable but wide and outwardly bulging lateral crura are transformed into disproportionately long, narrow, and flail crural remnants that can only achieve structural stability through concave collapse. The tendency to overresect the lateral crus has also been perpetuated by the misguided notion that a residual lateral crural width of 6.0 mm ensures adequate crural strength in virtually any nose. Although there is indeed a correlation between crural width and crural stability, width is only one of many physical determinants that govern crural stability. In addition to the shape-derived increases in support imparted by bulbous cupping and the nasal scroll, various other factors including cartilage thickness, cartilage stiffness, crural length, and secondary support mechanisms all combine to collectively determine crural stability and sidewall support. Hence the decision to resect crural cartilage must take into account not only the residual width of the lateral crus, but also its shape, length, and natural stiffness, and the all-important contributions of secondary support mechanisms. Although a cephalic trim can sometimes produce favorable long-term results in select individuals, even a modest cephalic resection can trigger deformity in the susceptible nose and determining exactly how much cartilage can be safely excised to enhance contour and avoid secondary deformity is virtually impossible. The uncertainty and the unprecedented morbidity associated with the cephalic trim create a strong incentive to abandon this risky and unpredictable procedure in favor of nonexcisional tip-refinement techniques.

SECONDARY TIP SUPPORT

The contribution of the LLC to intrinsic tip support is self-evident. However, secondary tip support, derived from the soft tissue and ligamentous interconnections of the LLC to neighboring skeletal components, is a less obvious, but nonetheless essential component of a strong and stable tip complex. As early as 1971, Janeke and Wright[12] published a landmark article defining the major tip support mechanisms of the nose. The authors identified four major areas where the LLC derive extrinsic support: (1) the nasal scroll, (2) the interdomal ligaments, (3) the attachments of the medial crura to the caudal septum, and (4) the sesamoid complex.[12] Likewise, the laminating effect of the inner and outer nasal lining, and the suspensory support of the nasal scroll ligament, are widely acknowledged as important sources of secondary tip support. The nasal septum is also a critical source of secondary tip support in most noses. Clinically, the contribution of the septum to secondary tip support is appreciated by observing the adverse effects of (dorsal) septal necrosis stemming from granulomatosis with polyangiitis (formerly known as Wegener granulomatosis), chronic cocaine abuse, or septal abscess formation. In fresh cadaver studies evaluating septal contributions to nasal tip support, dorsal septal resections of 4.0 mm performed through an open rhinoplasty approach produced a 3.3-mm average loss in tip projection despite intact LLC.[13] Moreover, complete resection of the cartilaginous septum resulted in a 3.6-mm average loss in tip projection, with losses up to 7.0 mm.[13] The authors concluded that septal support is likely equivalent to the LLC and their soft tissue attachments in providing structural support to the nasal tip. Without question, the contribution of septal undergirding is critical to tip stability in a large percentage of noses, and the importance of preserving adequate septal support should not be underestimated.

In summary, stable nasal tip support is a complex and fragile equilibrium that can diminish with disease, age, injury, and/or poorly executed nasal surgery. Given that surgery itself disrupts tip support to varying degrees, and that rhinoplasty is most often performed in early life, a concentrated effort to ensure robust structural tip support should be part of every rhinoplasty. Although natural tip support mechanisms are disrupted with the wide-field exposure of the external rhinoplasty approach, open rhinoplasty also facilitates structural fortification of the tip framework for unparalleled support and maximum long-term stability. Finally, the cephalic trim is no longer the exclusive means of achieving tip refinement because highly effective alternatives that preserve virtually the entire lateral crus are now available,[14] and the unprecedented morbidity of this destructive and haphazard procedure is now completely avoidable.

ALAR RIM SUPPORT

From a structural standpoint the caudal margin of the lateral crus provides a direct skeletal buttress that stabilizes the medial segment of the alar rim. In noses with naturally favorable alar contour, the lateral crus typically parallels the alar margin to near its midpoint at which point the crus then diverges superolaterally leaving the remaining nostril rim without direct skeletal support (**Fig. 2**). However, lateral to the divergence point the semirigid fibrous septae of tele subcutanea cutis serve to stiffen the alar lobule and assist in stabilizing lateral rim contour.[2,15] In natural noses with overly arched nostril rims, the divergence or "turning point" is

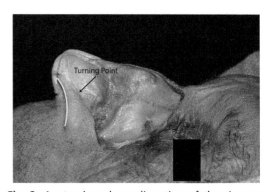

Fig. 2. Anatomic cadaver dissection of the tip complex. Note the favorable contour of the alar rim (*yellow line*) and the well-defined lateral crural "turning point" located at the mid-point of the alar rim (*arrow*). (*From* P. Ashley Wackym and James B. Snow Jr. C. 2016. Ballenger's Otorhinolaryngology Head and Neck Surgery, Vol 2, 18th ed., p. 732. Raleigh: PMPH-USA, Ltd; 2016.)

frequently displaced medially, or is poorly defined, or both, and thus the buttressing effect of the lateral crus is greatly diminished. Conversely, because a well-defined and laterally positioned divergence point enhances the buttressing effect along a greater portion of the nostril rim, congenital rim deformities, such as excessive arching, notching, or flaring, are far less common in this more favorable cartilage configuration.

PATHOPHYSIOLOGY OF IATROGENIC ALAR RETRACTION

Refinement of the nasal tip remains a highly challenging aspect of cosmetic rhinoplasty. The cephalic trim is a traditional and still widely used procedure directed at tip refinement that frequently, albeit inadvertently, destabilizes the tip complex. Arguably, the most problematic consequence of the cephalic trim is PSAR. Although other potential causes of iatrogenic alar retraction are possible, overresection of the lateral crus is almost always the root cause of PSAR.[4,8,9,11,16] Although traditional teaching recommends leaving a 6.0-mm remnant of crural cartilage to ensure structural stability, the average lateral crus is 12.0 mm in width,[3] and a 6.0-mm resection comprises approximately one-half of the lower sidewall framework.[17] Excising the upper half of the lateral crus also eliminates the shape-derived support provided by the nasal scroll, and a resection of this magnitude seldom leaves enough residual support for a favorable long-term result, especially in noses with naturally weak cartilage or contracture-prone soft tissues. In fresh cadaver studies conducted by Adams and colleagues[13] using the open rhinoplasty approach, an immediate 2.3-mm average loss in tip projection was observed simply by performing a cephalic trim with a 6.0-mm-wide rim strip. In addition to the potentially adverse impact on the nasal profile, tip deprojection also serves to increase sidewall laxity, thereby detensioning the surgically weakened lateral crural remnant and further increasing its vulnerability to upward retraction and inward collapse. The detensioning effect is perhaps most detrimental in the overprojected nose, in which cephalic resection leaves a narrow, flail, and sagging crural remnant that is far too long for the lower sidewall span. The result is a tremendous increase in sidewall laxity, which leaves the overly long and flaccid crural remnant highly susceptible to concave collapse and/or cephalic retraction.[16] This scenario is especially common in the bulbous tip complex because redundant crural length is intrinsic to cupped crural cartilages and the highly objectionable morphology (Fig. 1A) generates a strong temptation for overresection.

However, a surgically weakened lateral crus alone does not produce PSAR. Only when progressive epithelial contracture exerts sustained forces of deformation on the surgically weakened crural remnant does the upward displacement of PSAR occur. Because the amount of denuded epithelium determines the surface area contributing to epithelial contracture and the available space for crural displacement, and because the patient's nasal skin type and genetic predisposition determine the intensity of contracture acting on the surgically weakened crural remnant, a large skeletal void (ie, a narrow rim strip) in a thin-skinned and contracture-prone nose is far more likely to produce severe deformity. Collectively, the triad of (1) weak tip cartilage, (2) a large skeletal void with a narrow rim strip, and (3) thin contracture-prone skin, virtually guarantees severe PSAR from the synergistic interplay of these independent risk factors. Hence, it is not merely the width of the crural remnant, but rather the residual strength of the crural remnant, the size of the skeletal void, and the magnitude of forces acting to distort the remnant, that govern the ultimate degree of alar rim deformation. Crural overresection is often compounded by overresection of the septal L-strut with a loss of septal undergirding, which serves to exacerbate deprojection and overrotation of the tip complex, thereby further increasing sidewall laxity and predisposing to even greater alar rim distortion. In severe cases of PSAR, it is not uncommon to find crural remnants of only 2.0 to 3.0 mm in width (or even crura that are absent altogether) compounded by overresection of the caudal and/or dorsal segments of the quadrangular cartilage. Conversely, if cephalic resection is avoided, natural cartilage strength remains unaltered, no internal lining is denuded, and epithelial contracture is averted or negligible; and unless septal support is compromised and/or the central tip compartment is not adequately supported, PSAR is highly improbable. Ultimately, there is no way to determine with certainty what constitutes a safe and an effective cephalic trim. Accordingly, the cephalic trim should be regarded as a haphazard, potentially morbid, and unforgiving technique that is highly prone to delayed functional and cosmetic morbidity. In the opinion of the senior author (RED), cephalic resection should only be used judiciously and preferably not at all, especially because effective alternatives are now available.

SURGICAL TREATMENT STRATEGIES

Effective treatment of PSAR is exceedingly difficult because of (1) severe structural compromise of the lateral crus, (2) cicatricial contracture of the denuded vestibular lining and/or the overlying skin–soft tissue envelope, (3) fibrosis of the contractured and bunched vestibular lining resulting in severe inelasticity, and (4) adhesions between the inner and outer epithelial layers making subsequent dissection difficult. Historically, these impediments have proven difficult to overcome. In a retrospective review of 123 patients treated via the open rhinoplasty approach (including 73 secondary rhinoplasty patients) using adjunctive alar contour grafts (also known as alar rim grafts), Rohrich and coworkers[18] concluded that the alar contour graft is "very effective" for correcting mild to moderate alar retraction. However, the authors cited alar retraction caused by "scarring or lining loss" as the underlying cause of treatment failure in revision rhinoplasty cases, prompting them to advise against using alar contour grafts for PSAR with severe scarring. In a similar retrospective analysis of adjunctive alar rim grafts in 31 cases of cosmetic and functional rhinoplasty published by Boahene and Hilger,[19] the authors also advised against using alar rim grafts in moderate to severe cases of alar notching or alar retraction. As an alternative, composite grafts were advocated to overcome severe scarring or the loss of vestibular lining.[19]

LYSIS OF ADHESIONS AND RELEASE OF THE ALAR MARGIN

In this article we advocate a stepwise approach to the correction of PSAR using the principles of structural rhinoplasty. Before the crural-rim complex is successfully stabilized, adhesions incarcerating the malpositioned crural-rim complex must be eliminated to permit a tensionless release

and satisfactory repositioning of the alar rim. Using the external rhinoplasty approach, the outer nasal skin envelope is first carefully separated from the internal nasal lining to expose the entire cephalic border of the lateral crural remnant and the entire caudal border of the adjacent upper lateral cartilage (**Fig. 3**A). In severe cases, the two edges are in close approximation and densely scarred. Vestibular adhesions along the cephalic border of the crural remnant that restrict caudal movement are then carefully lysed while the alar rim is retracted caudally (**Fig. 3**B). Lysis of adhesions serves to progressively unfurl and lengthen the bunched and foreshortened vestibular lining, thereby releasing and downwardly mobilizing the crural-rim complex and simultaneously recreating the original skeletal void (**Fig. 3**C). Lysis of adhesions is tedious, and care must be taken not to injure the vestibular epithelium,[4,9,16] but a complete tension-free release using blunt dissection with or without partial thickness relaxing incisions (parallel to the caudal margin of the upper lateral cartilage) is exceedingly important and is performed in all cases to permit optimal repositioning of the alar rim. Although complete release of the crural-rim complex is not possible in every patient, with careful and painstaking dissection a return to normal, or near-normal alar rim position is possible in most instances, particularly if concomitant nasal lengthening or tip counterrotation are not also undertaken. Conversely, if adequate mobility of the crural-rim complex cannot be achieved through the lysis of adhesions, the approach to PSAR treatment described herein is unlikely to produce favorable results. Although (conchal) chondrocutaneous "composite grafts" are sometimes subject to ischemic failure, excessive thickness, and/or airway impingement, in cases of irreversible epithelial contracture or missing vestibular lining with an immobilized crural remnant, the use of

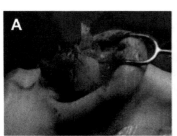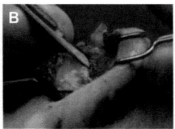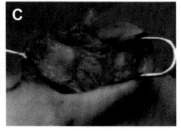

Fig. 3. Lysis of vestibular skin adhesions. (*A*) Initial exposure of the retracted lateral crural remnant with the open rhinoplasty approach. (*B*) Lysis of scar adhesions using partial-thickness vestibular skin incisions and downward retraction of the alar rim. (*C*) Full release of the crural remnant with recreation of the original skeletal void stemming from cephalic resection. Note significant downward movement of the crural-rim complex.

composite grafts remains the only viable treatment option for severe PSAR, and all patients should be consented for this possibility in advance.

RESTORING AND STABILIZING THE CENTRAL NASAL COMPARTMENT WITH THE SEPTAL EXTENSION GRAFT

Because severe PSAR most commonly occurs in noses that are also foreshortened, underprojected, and overrotated, restoring the size, shape, and strength of the septal L-strut is often the first step in the treatment of PSAR. However, even when the existing L-strut is straight, strong, and well-proportioned, additional support to the overresected tip complex is still required for effective treatment using this protocol. L-strut elongation, and/or stabilization of the overresected tip complex, are both best accomplished by means of a SEG.[20–24] When the L-strut/SEG construct lacks longitudinal stability, splinting grafts or extended spreader grafts are also used to ensure axial rigidity of the nasal "backbone," another critical requirement for the success of this protocol. A sturdy and stationary SEG not only augments L-strut length and establishes rigidity of the nasal axis, it also facilitates increases in tip projection and/or counterrotation of the tip complex (as needed), while simultaneously establishing a stationary "load-bearing wall" within the central tip compartment for reliable fixation of the repositioned LLC remnants. Creation of a midline and stationary load-bearing suspension wall then allows the application of longitudinal crural tensioning forces, which serve to reverse pathologic tip dynamics and facilitate effective long-term PSAR treatment.

Although achieving optimal nasal cosmesis often requires extending nasal length, elongation of the central tip compartment also projects the columella caudally, thus widening the gap separating the columella from the retracted alar rim. This not only worsens alar/columellar disharmony, it also increases the amount of alar rim movement needed to achieve a satisfactory alar/columellar relationship. In these challenging cases, restoration of ideal nasal length may need to be moderated unless alar rim movement can offset the large gap separating the alar rim and columella.

As with scar-mediated incarceration of the retracted crural-rim complex, nasal elongation may also be limited by scar-mediated inelasticity of the nasal skin envelope. Nasal elongation can prove difficult or even impossible unless soft tissue distensibility allows optimal skeletal elongation with minimal closing tension. Because excessive closing tension produces a corresponding increase in the forces of skeletal deformation and/or the risk of vascular insufficiency, the (cosmetically) ideal length of the skeletal framework may also require downsizing if skeletal deformation or vascular insufficiency threaten. Failure to maintain uninterrupted nutrient blood flow as a consequence of excessive closing tension and/or excessive swelling can lead to inadequate soft tissue perfusion with possible graft ischemia and/or compromised immune function with infection, and either complication can potentially lead to catastrophic treatment failure. Consequently, in all overresected and foreshortened noses, the risks of aggressive skeletal re-expansion must be carefully balanced against the desire for aesthetic optimization of the nose, and patients must be prewarned that compromises in ideal nasal length may become necessary to avoid catastrophic treatment failure.

Fortunately, in the motivated patient excessive closing tension is proactively avoided by increasing soft tissue distensibility. In the highly motivated patient who presents with a foreshortened nose, PSAR, and severely nondistensible skin, who also strongly desires aesthetic optimization, preoperative nasal skin-stretching exercises are used to gradually increase skin distensibility and thereby avoid excessive closing tension (**Fig. 4**). Skin stretching is performed by having the patient pull both nostrils in a downward and outward direction and maintaining vigorous stretch for 15 to 20 seconds (see **Fig. 4**F). This is followed by a 15- to 20-minute rest interval to prevent progressive inflammation. The process is then repeated throughout the day as tolerated. Stretching should be temporarily suspended if persistent erythema, pain, and swelling, or other signs of tissue intolerance develop. With regular and consistent skin-stretching, soft tissue distensibility increases incrementally over several months in a manner similar to tissue expansion. By pulling both retracted nostril rims simultaneously, the lateral nasal compartments are being mobilized in unison so that each crural-rim complex becomes more downwardly distensible. When columellar retraction is also present, the columellar skin can also be stretched independently for uniform lengthening of the central and lateral compartments. Surgically elongating a foreshortened and contractured nose with PSAR and nondistensible skin is one of the most daunting challenges in aesthetic nasal surgery, but in the highly motivated patient successful preoperative skin-stretching can become the difference between treatment success and failure[25] (see **Fig. 4**K–N). When applied diligently and properly, stretching exercises alone eventually begin to release and caudally reposition the retracted

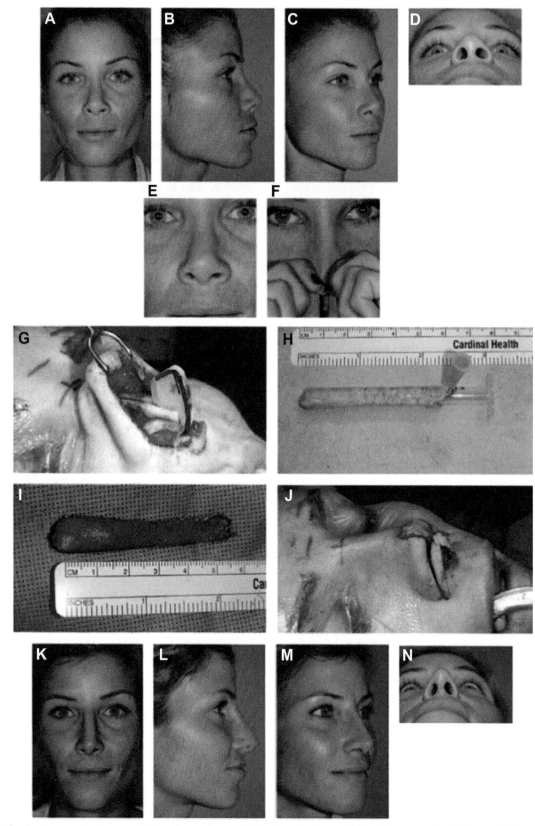

Fig. 4. Overresected nose with foreshortening and fibrotic inelastic nasal skin. Pre-operative (*A*) frontal, (*B*) profile, (*C*) oblique, and (*D*) base views showing overly short overrotated nose with upwardly retracted nostril rims.

crural-rim complex thereby greatly improving the prognosis for mobilization and effective surgical stabilization of the alar rim. However, without the direct skeletal support provided by the AARG and advocated in this treatment paradigm, the likelihood of permanent correction is low because retraction will likely recur on cessation of skin-stretching exercises. Finally, patient expectations should always be carefully tempered in the foreshortened nose with PSAR because even a sturdy skeletal frame may not prevent the ill-effects of severe and sustained shrink-wrap contracture in every nose. However, if postoperative swelling and contracture begin to upwardly displace the alar margin, gentle resumption of skin-stretching exercises can often be used to salvage the surgical outcome.

RE-ENGINEERING TIP DYNAMICS TO RESIST RECURRENT POSTSURGICAL ALAR RETRACTION WITH LATERAL CRURAL TENSIONING

As the overresected nose progressively shrinks and contracts, buttressing support from the weakened lateral crus is rendered increasingly ineffective, and unopposed upward arching or notching of the crural-rim complex ensues. However, by using a SEG to establish rigid midline tip support, tip contour is optimized and the crural-rim complex can also be securely stabilized after its release. By contouring the outer silhouette of the SEG to reflect the desired tip profile, a discrete and well-defined tip-defining point (TDP) is created (**Fig. 5**), which can be positioned to simultaneously guide correction of deficiencies in tip rotation and/or tip projection. In this manner, the SEG becomes a perfectly shaped and ideally positioned scaffold for cosmetically optimized resuspension and fixation of the weakened crural-rim complex (**Figs. 1E, 6A**). Because the SEG also serves as a stationary load-bearing wall hidden within the central tip compartment, it can also withstand tensioning forces generated by stretching the crural remnant between its piriform attachments laterally, and the SEG/TDP medially.[11,14,16] However, to prevent excessive tension and potential instability, crural length must first be adjusted to match the newly

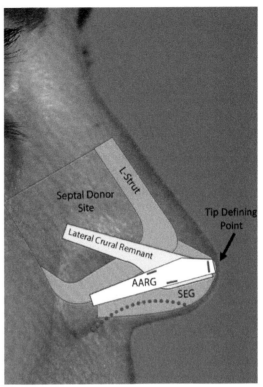

Fig. 5. Schematic overlay showing SEG and AARG placement. Note position of the AARG relative to the SEG/TDP, the newly repositioned alar rim (*dotted red line*), the lateral crural remnant, and the (*central*) alar lobule. Also, note the three AARG fixation points (*solid red lines*) at the TDP, the crural "turning point," and the lateral-most junction of the AARG with the crural remnant.

altered sidewall span. In most instances, length adjustments are accomplished via relocation of the domal fold along the LLC, either laterally in the case of redundant crural length, or medially in the case of inadequate crural length, so that suture fixation of the newly created crural dome (**Fig. 1F**) generates modest longitudinal crural tension that tightens, lifts, flattens, and stiffens the remnant cartilage. In doing so, tip dynamics are re-engineered to reduce laxity within the entire tip sidewall, enhance sidewall contour, increase resting sidewall tone, and dramatically strengthen the tip framework, all without bulky sidewall grafts

(*E*) frontal and (*F*) frontal stretched nose views of difference in skin distensibility after 5 months of skin-stretching exercises. Intra-operative views of (*G*) extended spreader graft and septal extension graft placement, (*H*) fabrication of the temporalis fascia sleeve, (*I*) the assembled diced rib cartilage – fascia (DC-F) graft, and (*J*) the in situ DC-F graft and reconstructed tip complex. Corresponding postoperative (*K*) frontal, (*L*) profile (*M*) oblique, and (*N*) base views demonstrating marked improvement in alar rim contour despite extensive increases in nasal length and tip projection. (*From* Davis R, Hrisomalos E. Surgical Management of the Thick-Skinned Nose. *Facial Plast Surg.* 2018;34(01):22-28.)

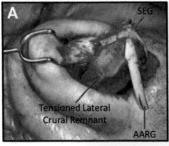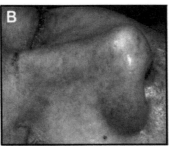

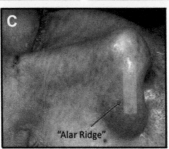

Fig. 6. Open revision rhinoplasty using rib cartilage. (A) Intraoperative view showing the SEG, the tensioned lateral crural remnant, and the AARG. (B) External nasal contour after skin closure. (C) Note aesthetically favorable accentuation of the "alar ridge" after AARG placement.

or unwanted rotation of the tip complex. The final result of LCT is a thin and flat, yet taut and sturdy lower nasal sidewall that corrects concave collapse and eliminates residual tip bulbosity while also resisting upward rim displacement and dynamic nasal valve collapse. Reconfiguration of tip dynamics with LCT is a critical second step in reshaping and stabilizing the formerly malpositioned and misshapen crural-rim complex. Without the biomechanical benefits of LCT to oppose the unremitting forces of contracture, the likelihood of long-term success is low. However, when LCT is performed bilaterally in a judicious and balanced fashion, and stabilized by secure suture fixation, a strong, stable, and resilient tip complex is created that mimics nature and simultaneously optimizes form and function in virtually any misshapen nose.[14,16]

PROVIDING DIRECT ALAR RIM SUPPORT WITH THE ARTICULATED ALAR RIM GRAFT

The final step in PSAR correction is AARG placement. In severe cases of PSAR, AARG placement without the tandem benefits of LCT (made possible by the stationary support of the SEG), would likely prove ineffective. Conversely, the combined use of LCT and AARG placement are complimentary and thus far more effective. The AARG is a modification of the conventional alar rim graft/alar contour graft that provides direct skeletal support to the entire crural-rim complex via rigid integration into the tip framework.[16] As with virtually any structural graft, its long-term efficacy is dependent on its rigidity, proper

fabrication, secure fixation, and long-term survival, and individuals with naturally weak donor cartilage and/or strong shrink-wrap tendencies are more prone to graft failure.

Previously, we have demonstrated clinical efficacy in the correction of PSAR using our treatment protocol with the AARG.[16] In a retrospective evaluation of clinical outcomes in 47 consecutive patients undergoing combined SEG placement, LCT, and AARG placement (in primary and secondary rhinoplasty with a mean follow-up of 7 months), total correction of moderate to severe PSAR (with or without lobular pinching) was observed in 11 of 17 patients (65%) and substantial improvement was observed in the remaining six patients.[16] Eight secondary rhinoplasty patients treated for lobular and/or supra-alar pinching also demonstrated total correction at follow-up. In five secondary rhinoplasty patients treated for external valve collapse, two patients demonstrated complete correction, two patients demonstrated partial correction, and one patient failed treatment. Hence, using the protocol described herein, alar deformities were completely eliminated in 70% of secondary rhinoplasty patients, substantially improved in 27% of secondary rhinoplasty patients, and unsuccessful (3%) in one secondary rhinoplasty patient with severe external valve collapse. All primary rhinoplasty patients who were treated for mild congenital deformities, such as excessive alar arching or alar notching, also demonstrated favorable outcomes at follow-up. Furthermore, at a mean follow-up of

7 months, there were no overly visible grafts, graft displacements, graft infections, or graft extrusions observed; and no patients voiced complaints relating to AARG placement.

To optimize efficacy, proper AARG fabrication, placement, and fixation are essential. Unlike the commonly used lateral crural strut graft, which is an underlayment graft, the AARG is placed on the superficial surface of the crural remnant to accentuate the alar ridge[16] (see **Fig. 5**). Moreover, it does not parallel the crural remnant, rather it diverges caudally to buttress the entire nostril margin. For optimal effectiveness, the AARG must be a rigid strip of autologous cartilage, preferably fabricated from septal or rib cartilage for its greater stability. Although graft shape must be individualized to accommodate individual variations in tip contour and to ensure tip symmetry, the typical graft measures approximately 22.0 to 25.0 mm in length, 4.0 to 5.0 mm in greatest width, and approximately 1.5 to 2.0 mm in thickness. It is also tapered at both ends, beveled along its cephalic and medial borders for concealment, and is either flat or slightly convex (**Fig. 6**). Because the AARG is meant to provide direct skeletal support along the entire alar rim, it should originate at the TDP (flush with the most projecting point of the SEG), and then parallel the alar rim where it ends in the central aspect of the alar lobule. The efficacy of the AARG is only as good as its stability. Secure three-point fixation is achieved using 4–0 or 5–0 polydioxanone mattress sutures to the underlying crural remnant and to the adjacent SEG (see **Fig. 5**). The first fixation point is medially at the TDP, where the suture is first passed (from the contralateral side) through the SEG and intervening ipsilateral dome, and then back. This fixation point is critical because it anchors the AARG to the most projecting point of the tip lobule for optimal alignment of the alar ridge, and it structurally unites the AARG with the septal L-strut for maximum stability. Two additional 4–0 or 5–0 polydioxanone mattress sutures are then placed between the AARG and the underlying crural remnant. The first suture is placed along the caudal margin of the AARG beside the divergence point, and the second mattress suture is placed on the cephalic margin of the AARG where it diverges from the crural remnant laterally. Following fixation, a skin pocket is often created to accommodate the graft lateral to the marginal incision. A tapered skin pocket is dissected superficially along the alar ridge (approximately 2 mm above the alar margin), beginning medially at the marginal incision and extending laterally to the central aspect of the

alar lobule. The alar lobule is then retracted laterally to facilitate gentle insertion of the AARG into the skin pocket. However, if the marginal incision can be closed loosely without a skin pocket, this is preferable because it will stabilize the entire alar lobule from above. The need for a skin pocket, the location of the skin pocket, and the graft size and shape vary according to the specific contour irregularities of the crural rim complex and the nasal tip, and AARG treatment must be individualized for optimal results.

DISCUSSION

Herein we present a step-wise approach for treatment of PSAR predicated on complete release of the retracted alar rim, followed by stabilization of the newly repositioned crural-rim complex. This protocol seeks not only to eliminate crural entrapment by disrupting adhesions and contractures, but also to eliminate crural laxity, crural length discrepancies, excessive crural pliability, and any losses in secondary tip support that allowed shrink-wrap contracture to distort the crural remnant. No one single component of this protocol is likely to succeed in isolation, but when applied in concert, the probability of a satisfactory outcome is high.

The first step in this protocol is achieving a tensionless release and mobilization of the incarcerated crural-rim complex through the lysis of adhesions. Unless the alar rim can be favorably repositioned without vertical tension, the remaining steps in the paradigm will most likely fail or provide only partial correction. Carefully unfurling the contractured and fibrosed vestibular lining is tedious, but painstaking dissection using parallel relaxing incisions via the open rhinoplasty approach is most often successful (see **Fig. 3**). If complete release is not possible, composite graft placement is needed to replace lost vestibular lining, but the biomechanical and architectural advantages of LCT are still valid, and LCT is recommended regardless of how the lateral crus is freed.

The remaining steps in this protocol are then aimed at stabilization of the newly mobilized crural-rim complex. Placement of a SEG is fundamental to this treatment paradigm because it must counteract the loading forces transmitted by LCT and AARG placement. Likewise, without LCT and AARG placement, recurrent alar retraction is virtually inevitable because the forces of cicatricial contracture remain unopposed. Hence, all three stabilization maneuvers are critical to success, and the efficacy of each maneuver depends on the contribution of the other two.

The numerous benefits of LCT are often misunderstood and underappreciated. Because LCT serves to longitudinally stretch and flatten the crural remnant, it not only generates tensioning forces that oppose recurrent retraction, it also eliminates crural concavity and/or residual tip bulbosity for a better nasal contour. And because LCT enhances nasal contour by improving sidewall tone, position, and rigidity, in most cases it will also increase internal nasal valve dimensions and simultaneously raise the threshold for dynamic valve collapse. LCT also avoids the problematic bulk and weight associated with lateral crural batten grafts or traditional lateral crural strut grafts that frequently narrow the internal valve aperture and simultaneously lower the threshold for dynamic valve collapse.

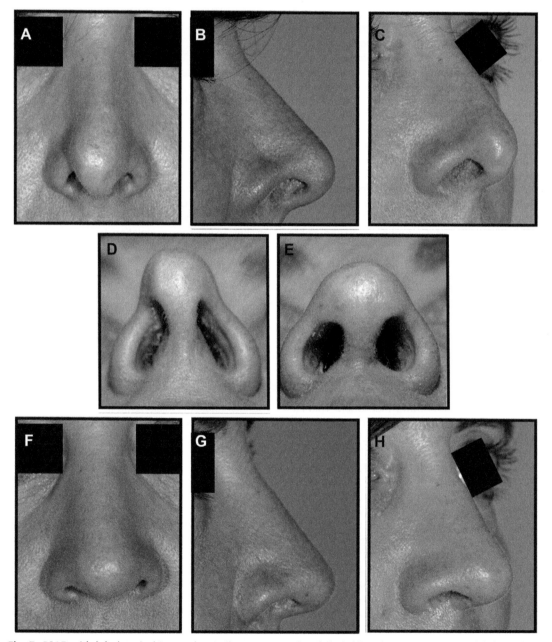

Fig. 7. PSAR with lobular pinching and nostril asymmetry after failed rhinoplasty. Preoperative (*A*) frontal, (*B*) profile, (*C*) oblique, and (*D*) base views showing iatrogenic crural overresection with aesthetic and functional morbidity. Corresponding postoperative (*E*) base, (*F*) frontal, (*G*) profile, and (*H*) oblique views showing improved function and tip contour despite nasal elongation.

The final step of this protocol is AARG placement. The AARG is a structurally integrated alar rim graft that enjoys all the same benefits of the conventional (floating) alar rim graft in primary rhinoplasty applications, including satisfactory prophylaxis against postsurgical rim distortion and/or the elimination of most congenital rim deformities. However, the AARG is also uniquely well-suited to the correction of acquired alar rim deformities, particularly PSAR, and in our hands the elimination or substantial improvement of surgically acquired rim deformities was largely complication free.[16] Moreover, the cosmetic benefits of the AARG are many. When the healthy and attractive nose is viewed from the front, the light reflex generated by the TDP is horizontally aligned with the central aspect of the adjacent alar lobules. In the attractive nose the TDP also transitions seamlessly to the alar lobule via a flat, straight, and narrow ridgeline located approximately 2.0 mm cephalad to the alar rim[26] that we have previously termed the "alar ridge"[16] (see **Fig. 6**C). Various cosmetic disturbances, congenital and acquired, such as a highly arched nostril rim, lobular pinching, alar retraction, alar notching, alar collapse, or nostril asymmetry, disrupt the smooth, flat, and straight contour of the alar ridge causing distortions in alar rim shape, fullness, and/or symmetry that range from subtle to severe. Because the AARG reconstitutes alar ridge support using an autologous, nonanatomic graft that is stabilized by integration into the tip framework, the fullness, linearity, shape, and symmetry of the alar ridges are typically restored.[14,16] Although the AARG has not supplanted the occasional need for chondrocutaneous composite grafts in cases of vestibular skin necrosis or severe epithelial scarring, this safe and effective modification of the conventional alar rim graft has proven to be a reliable workhorse in the rehabilitation of most iatrogenic alar rim deformities, especially PSAR (**Fig. 7**). Moreover, accentuation of the alar ridge with AARG placement is aesthetically pleasing in virtually any nose; and when combined with LCT, airway patency is safeguarded and overall airway function is typically improved.

REFERENCES

1. Holden P, Liaw L, Wong B. Human nasal cartilage ultrastructure: characteristics and comparison using scanning electron microscopy. Laryngoscope 2008;118:1153–6.
2. Patel J, Fletcher J, Singer D, et al. An anatomic and histologic analysis of the alar-facial crease and the lateral crus. Ann Plast Surg 2004;52:371–4.
3. Hatzis G, Sherry S, Hogan G, et al. Observations of the marginal incision and lateral crura alar cartilage assymetry in rhinoplasty: a fixed cadaver study. Oral Surg Oral Med Oral Pathol Oral Radiol Endod 2004;97(4):432–7.
4. Davis R. Revision of the over-resected tip complex. Facial Plast Surg 2012;28(4):427–39.
5. Kinkade K. What would it take to build a completely tornado-proof house? Forbes Mag 2016. Available at: https://www.forbes.com/sites/quora/2016/03/22/what-would-it-take-to-build-a-completely-tornado-proof-house/#6ee311c727ca.
6. Hamidpour R, Graham D. Prevention plan to save human life, by building safe monolithic dome or ecoshell structures. J Civ Environ Eng 2014;4(4):153.
7. Hiroshima Peace Memorial (Genbaku Dome). UNESCO World Heritage Convention. Available at: https://whc.unesco.org/en/list/775. Accessed March 11, 2019.
8. Gubisch W, Eichhorn-Sens J. Overresection of the lower lateral cartilages: a common conceptual mistake with functional and aesthetic consequences. Aesthetic Plast Surg 2009;33(1):6–13.
9. Davis RE. Nasal tip complications. Facial Plast Surg 2012;28(3):294–302.
10. Davis R, Bublik M. Common technical causes of the failed rhinoplasty. Facial Plast Surg 2012;28(4):380–9.
11. Davis R. Revision rhinoplasty. In: Johnson J, Rosen C, editors. Bailey's head and neck surgery - otolaryngology. 5th edition. Philadelphia: Wolters Kluwer/Lippincott Williams & Wilkins; 2014. p. 2989–3052.
12. Janeke JB, Wright WK. Studies on the support of the nasal tip. Arch Otolaryngol 1971;93(5):458–64.
13. Adams WP, Rohrich RJ, Hollier LH, et al. Anatomic basis and clinical implications for nasal tip support in open versus closed rhinoplasty. Plast Reconstr Surg 1999;103(1):255–61.
14. Davis R. Lateral crural tensioning for refinement of the wide and underprojected nasal tip: rethinking the lateral crural steal. Facial Plast Surg Clin North Am 2015;23(1):23–53.
15. Daniel R, Glasz T, Molnar G, et al. The lower nasal base: an anatomical study. Aesthet Surg J 2013;33(2):222–32.
16. Ballin A, Kim H, Chance E, et al. The articulated alar rim graft: reengineering the conventional alar rim graft for improved contour and support. Facial Plast Surg 2016;32:384–97.
17. Gruber R, Chang E, Buchanan E. Suture techniques in rhinoplasty. Clin Plast Surg 2010;37(2):231–43.
18. Rohrich R, Raniere JJ, Ha R. The alar contour graft: correction and prevention of alar rim deformities in rhinoplasty. Plast Reconstr Surg 2002;109(7):2495–505.

19. Boahene K, Hilger PA. Alar rim grafting in rhinoplasty: indications, technique, and outcomes. Arch Facial Plast Surg 2009;11(5):285–9.

20. Toriumi D. Caudal septal extension graft for correction of the retracted columella. Oper Tech Otolaryngol-Head Neck Surg 1995;6(4): 311–8. Available at: https://www.sciencedirect.com/science/article/abs/pii/S1043181005800089.

21. Naficy S, Baker S. Lengthening the short nose. Arch Otolaryngol Head Neck Surg 1998;124: 809–13.

22. Ha R, Byrd H. Septal extension grafts revisited: 6-year experience in controlling nasal tip projection and shape. Plast Reconstr Surg 2003;112(7): 1929–35.

23. Guyuron B, Varghai A. Lengthening the nose with a tongue-and groove technique. Plast Reconstr Surg 2003;111(4):1533–9.

24. Byrd H, Andochick S, Copit S, et al. Septal extension grafts: a method of controlling tip projection shape. Plast Reconstr Surg 1997;100(4):999–1010.

25. Davis R, Hrisomalos E. Surgical management of the thick-skinned nose. Facial Plast Surg 2018;34(1):22–8.

26. Toriumi D. New concepts in nasal tip contouring. Arch Facial Plast Surg 2006;8(3):156–85.

Treatment Protocol for Compromised Nasal Skin

Julia L. Kerolus, MD[a],*, Paul S. Nassif, MD, FACS[b]

KEYWORDS

- Skin necrosis • Thinned nasal skin • Nasal skin–soft tissue envelope • Vascular compromise
- Revision rhinoplasty • Treatment protocol • Leeches • Hyperbaric oxygen

KEY POINTS

- Skin compromise after rhinoplasty can occur from aggressive thinning of the nasal skin–soft tissue envelope, infection, and vascular compression from excess tension on the skin.
- An understanding of the nasal soft tissue anatomy and corresponding vascular supply is paramount for achieving the optimal aesthetic results as well as preventing complications.
- Recognition of risk factors for vascular compromise and careful implementation of preventative measures in the perioperative period can decrease the development of skin necrosis.
- The treatment protocol for devascularized nasal skin includes the application of topical nitroglycerin, use of hyperbaric oxygen, leech therapy, a variety of medications, and regular follow-up visits.

INTRODUCTION

Complex nasal anatomy and unpredictable healing make rhinoplasty one of the most challenging operations that plastic surgeons perform. In addition to the complicated nature of the operation, patient dissatisfaction after surgery is not uncommon. Although not life-threatening, the perceived negative cosmetic outcome often leads patients to seek revision surgery.[1]

Secondary rhinoplasty carries additional challenges for the surgeon and frequently increased risk to the patient. Nasal skin compromise is a rare but devastating complication of both primary and revision rhinoplasty. It can occur as a result of lengthening the short nose, augmentation rhinoplasty, aggressive thinning of the skin–soft tissue envelope, infection, and history of prior filler injection. There have been several published articles regarding the treatment of impending necrosis after injection of dermal filler[2]; however, none describes management of compromised nasal skin after rhinoplasty. The authors describe experience with recognition, treatment, and prevention of nasal skin compromise after rhinoplasty.

NASAL SKIN ENVELOPE

The quality of the nasal skin is a significant predictor of surgical outcome and should be carefully considered in preoperative planning. The nasal skin–soft tissue envelope is composed of fat, muscle, overlying superficial musculoaponeurotic system (SMAS), and skin.[3] These layers can all vary in thickness and quality based on age, gender, and ethnicity.[4] There also are substantial differences in skin thickness and sebaceous gland activity within the different nasal subunits in each individual. Generally, the skin is thickest in the radix and supratip areas and thinnest at the rhinion.[5] The caudal half of the nose contains a higher density of sebaceous glands compared with the cephalic half.

Just deep to the skin lies the subcutaneous tissue composed of fat and fibroconnective tissue ligaments that anchor the overlying dermis to the

[a] Department of Otolaryngology–Head and Neck Surgery, Division of Facial Plastic and Reconstructive Surgery, University of Illinois at Chicago-College of Medicine, 1855 W Taylor Street Suite 2.42 (MC 648), Chicago, IL 60612, USA; [b] Nassif MD, Inc. and Associates, 120 South Spalding Drive Suite 301, Beverly Hills, CA 90212, USA
* Corresponding author.
E-mail address: jfrisend@uic.edu

Facial Plast Surg Clin N Am 27 (2019) 505–511
https://doi.org/10.1016/j.fsc.2019.07.007

deeper SMAS layer. The SMAS encapsulates the mimetic muscles of the face that insert onto the nasal structures. These muscles include the procerus, levator labii superioris alaeque nasi, dilator naris, compressor naris, and depressor septi. The blood supply to the skin relies on perforating vessels of the subdermal plexus that originate from the facial and ophthalmic arteries.[6] Vascular compression of these smaller vessels is possible in the tip and over the dorsum after augmentation of these areas in rhinoplasty. Open rhinoplasty interrupts the columellar artery blood supply, further increasing the risk to the skin.

Surgeons are faced with a challenge when patients presenting for reductive rhinoplasty are also plagued with thick nasal skin. Guyuron and Lee[7] describe several techniques to address the thick skin–soft tissue envelope in patients undergoing rhinoplasty. They advocate for raising a thick skin flap with subsequent removal of the deep fibrofatty tissue in the supratip area and between the domes. This technique is often misunderstood and the surgeon proceeds with thinning of the SMAS and subcutaneous fat rather than the sub-SMAS fat. This can lead to interruption of blood supply and irregular skin contraction after surgery. Equally as problematic is patients with very thin or scarred skin in which the dermis is densely adherent to the underling nasal structure. In these patients, a submucoperichondrial dissection off the nasal skeleton maintains vascular integrity and prevents violation of the skin.

RISK FACTORS

Surgeons must be additionally mindful in patients with risk factors for skin compromise. These include nicotine use, history of prior radiation therapy, rhinoplasty or nasal dermal filler injection in the past, prior foreign body placement (synthetic graft or filler), cocaine use, and thin or scarred nasal skin. Patients with systemic diseases, such as diabetes mellitus and granulomatosis with polyangiitis (formerly known as Wegener's granulomatosis), carry even greater risk.

TREATMENT PROTOCOL

The treatment of skin compromise after rhinoplasty is time sensitive. Immediate recognition and rapid implementation of the following measures can decrease the risk of necrosis and resulting tissue loss. Evidence of skin compromise is often evident once the initial transcolumellar skin sutures are placed (**Fig. 1**). Once recognized, the first step involves application of a thin layer of topical nitroglycerin 2% ointment (Nitro-Bid,

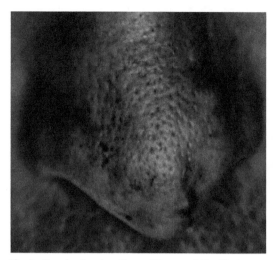

Fig. 1. Purple discoloration of the nasal tip skin immediately on closure of the transcolumellar incision.

Fougera Pharmaceuticals, Melville, New York) to the area of concern (**Fig. 2**). The authors use a dose of less than 7.5 mg per application. Care must be taken to avoid excess use of topical nitroglycerin given the risk for systemic hypotension or severe headache. The ointment is applied twice daily for the next several days. The patient is counseled on potential side effects, including application site irritation, erythema, edema, papules, and dermal thickening. These effects resolve with cessation of the medication. Because the use of topical nitroglycerin for treatment of vascular skin compromise is off-label, this also must be disclosed to the patient.[8]

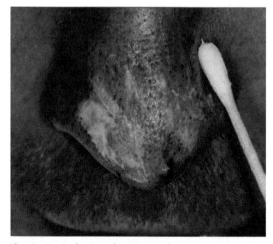

Fig. 2. Topical nitroglycerin application in the operating room prior to extubation. The amount is limited to a thin layer to prevent systemic hypotension and the blood pressure is monitored carefully.

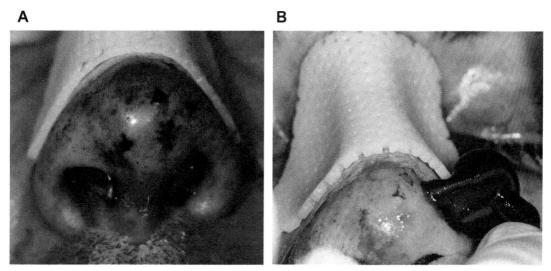

Fig. 3. (*A*) Before and (*B*) during medical-grade leech therapy on postoperative day 1. Note the significant improvement in skin color once the leech has latched.

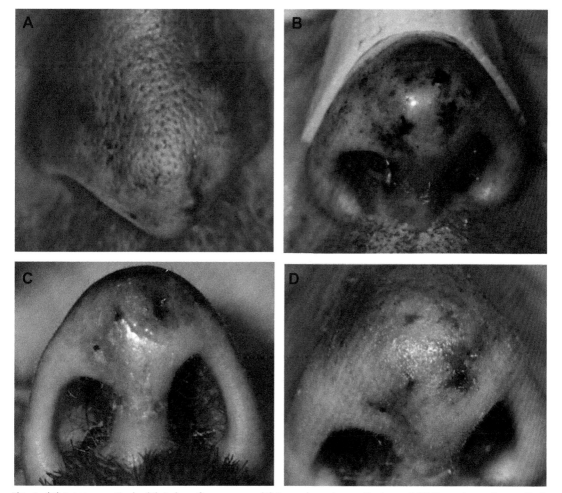

Fig. 4. (*A*) Intraoperatively, (*B*) 1 day after surgery, (*C*) 1 week postoperatively, and (*D*) 2 weeks postoperatively after the use of topical nitroglycerin, medicinal leeches, hyperbaric oxygen, and oral and intranasal antibiotics.

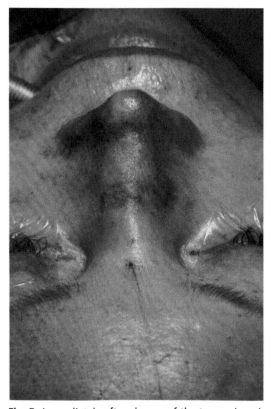

Fig. 5. Immediately after closure of the transcolumellar incision.

Leech therapy is used depending on the level of concern and risk for tissue loss (**Fig. 3**). Prophylaxis with oral ciprofloxacin or trimethoprim-sulfamethoxazole is required when using medicinal leeches to prevent infection with *Aeromonas hydrophila*.[9] Given the efficacy of leech therapy in treatment of vascular congestion, the authors now use leeches in the immediate postoperative period in patients with concern for potential necrosis, rather than waiting until the first or second postoperative day.

Patients are usually sent for daily hyperbaric oxygen dives and instructed to take oral aspirin, 81 mg daily. The authors recommend patients on aspirin also take an antacid to prevent the development of peptic bleeding or ulcer formation. Prophylactic antibiotics are started at the earliest sign of skin compromise. If overt infection does develop, culture-directed therapy is pursued, and infectious disease consult is sought. Oral antibiotics usually consist of ciprofloxacin and trimethoprim-sulfamethoxazole with the addition of topical intranasal mupirocin ointment twice daily. **Fig. 4** demonstrates the progression of a patient who was treated with this protocol. He has no long-term sequalae 2 years after his operation.

In severe cases, patients are given pentoxifylline, 400 mg, 2 times to 3 times per day. Pentoxifylline is a vasodilator that also reduces blood viscosity and improves peripheral tissue oxygenation.[10] If necrosis does develop, patients apply topical collagenase ointment once daily to the necrotic areas only. This serves to débride collagen in necrotic tissue. Collagenase is applied until débridement is complete. Patients with necrosis are treated with the addition of pentoxifylline and topical collagenase ointment (**Figs. 5–10**).

With any complication, consistent communication and regular in-person follow-up visits are critical. In impending skin necrosis, identification of progression or response to treatment is required to appropriately guide next steps. This includes

A

B

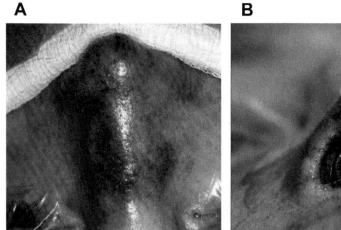
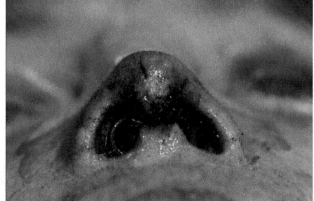

Fig. 6. (*A*) Frontal and (*B*) base views demonstrating the rapid progression of skin compromise during this patient's second operation.

A

B

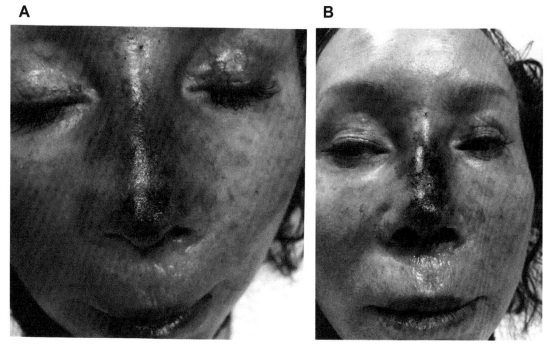

Fig. 7. (*A*) Postoperative day 1 showing skin compromise over the bridge and tip. (*B*) Postoperative day 2 with further progression and eschar formation over the tip.

several in-person visits per week for several weeks.

PREVENTION

Various strategies can be employed to prevent nasal skin necrosis after surgery. Control of comorbidities preoperatively can significantly decrease the likelihood of skin compromise after rhinoplasty. Patients with history of nicotine use should be counseled on the additional risk this carries for wound breakdown and skin necrosis. Smokers are instructed to avoid all nicotine

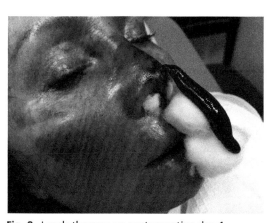

Fig. 8. Leech therapy on postoperative day 1.

products (including gum and patches) at least 6 weeks prior to surgery and continue to abstain throughout their recovery. If there is question of compliance, the authors advocate a urine nicotine test be administered prior to any surgical intervention.

Similarly, patients with a history of multiple prior nasal surgeries or previous dermal filler injections to the nose should be counseled regarding potential for postoperative complications. Preoperative hyperbaric oxygen therapy should be considered in smokers, patients who have had multiple prior surgeries, and those with a history of prior skin compromise.

During operative planning, thick nasal skin should be noted and, depending on the layer contributing to the thickness, addressed either before or during surgery. The surgeon can drastically decrease the risk of skin compromise by appropriately addressing the skin envelope. If skin thickness is primarily secondary to increased density of sebaceous structures, the surgeon may consider dermatologic referral for treatment with topical retinoids or oral isotretinoin because aggressive thinning of the SMAS have only a detrimental effect in these patients.[7,11] Patients with increased dermal thickness do not respond to skin care regimens and must be treated with various surgical maneuvers. Removal of sub-SMAS fibrofatty tissue between the domes and

A   B

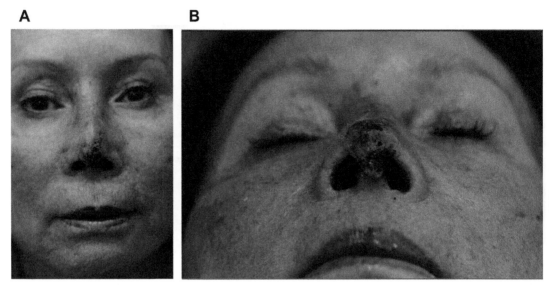

Fig. 9. (*A*) Frontal and (*B*) base views on postoperative day 5. Patient underwent treatment with topical nitroglycerin, medicinal leeches, hyperbaric oxygen, topical collagenase, pentoxyphylline, aspirin 81 mg, and antibiotics.

at the supratip aids in decreasing fullness in these areas. Eliminating dead space with a subcutaneous suture at the supratip and resecting redundant envelope help improve skin contraction postoperatively without increasing risk of vascular injury. In patients with thin or scarred skin, the authors advocate a submucoperichondrial dissection to preserve vascular integrity.

A   B

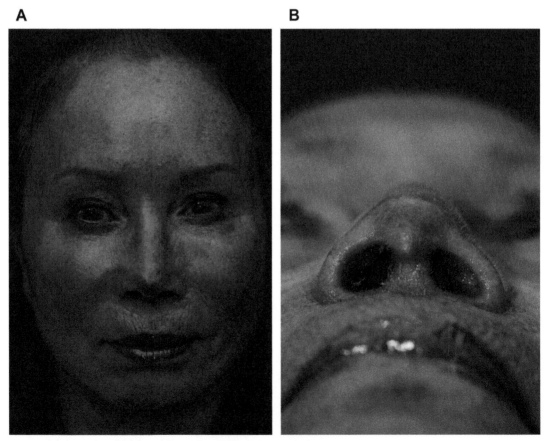

Fig. 10. (*A*) Frontal and (*B*) base views 4 months postoperatively.

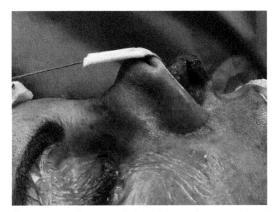

Fig. 11. Use of cotton pledget for gentle retraction of the skin envelope. Removed regularly to allow for vascular inflow.

Once the skin envelope has been elevated, the authors have found it helpful to gently retract the nasal skin with a cottonoid (**Fig. 11**) and let this down periodically throughout the operation to prevent venous congestion or arterial compression. The authors avoid the use of electrocautery in surgery because most bleeding can be controlled with injection of epinephrine locally and with pressure.

It may be prudent to avoid nasal taping and casting postoperatively. This allows for close monitoring of the skin envelope and avoids additional external compression (see **Fig. 6**). If casting is needed, some investigators advocate use of a thermoplastic nasal splint rather than a metallic split because this may be more forgiving. Similarly, the use of Doyle splints or intranasal packing should be avoided in patients with evidence of skin compromise. Use of postoperative oral antibiotics is recommended in patients undergoing complex rhinoplasty or revision surgery.[12]

SUMMARY

Skin compromise after rhinoplasty can lead to irreversible tissue loss and permanent deformity. Early recognition and prompt treatment can drastically decrease the risk of permanent sequelae. Therapies, such as topical nitroglycerin, medicinal leeches, hyperbaric oxygen, antibiotics, and

vasodilatory medications, all can aid in prevention of necrosis. Preoperative counseling and risk assessment for skin compromise are vital when considering primary or revision rhinoplasty.

REFERENCES

1. Neaman KC, Boettcher AK, Do VH, et al. Cosmetic rhinoplasty: revision rates revisited. Aesthet Surg J 2013;33(1):31–7.
2. Cohen JL, Biesman BS, Dayan SH, et al. Treatment of hyaluronic acid filler-induced impending necrosis with hyaluronidase: consensus recommendations. Aesthet Surg J 2015;35(7):844–9.
3. Ozturk CN, Larson JD, Ozturk C, et al. The SMAS and fat compartments of the nose: an anatomical study. Aesthetic Plast Surg 2013;37(1):11–5.
4. Kosins AM, Obagi ZE. Managing the difficulty soft tissue envelope in facial and rhinoplasty surgery. Aesthet Surg J 2017;37(2):143–57.
5. Cho GS, Kim JH, Yeo NK, et al. Nasal skin thickness measured using computed tomography and its effect on tip surgery outcomes. Otolaryngol Head Neck Surg 2011;114(4):522–7.
6. Saban Y, Amodeo AC, Douaziz D. Nasal arterial vasculature: medical and surgical applications. Arch Facial Plast Surg 2012;14(6):429–36.
7. Guyuron B, Lee M. An effective algorithm for management of noses with thick skin. Aesthetic Plast Surg 2017;41(2):381–7.
8. Kleydman K, Cohen JL, Marmur E. Nitroglycerin: a review of its use in the treatment of vascular occlusion after soft tissue augmentation. Dermatol Surg 2012;38(12):1889–97.
9. Kruer RM, Barton CA, Roberti G, et al. Antimicrobial Prophylaxis during Hirudo medicinalis therapy: a multicenter study. J Reconstr Microsurg 2015; 31(3):205–9.
10. Ahmadi M, Khalili H. Potential benefits of pentoxifylline on wound healing. Expert Rev Clin Pharmacol 2016;9(1):129–42.
11. Cobo R, Vitery L. Isotretinoin use in thick-skinned rhinoplasty patients. Facial Plast Surg 2016;32(6): 656–61.
12. Kullar R, Frisenda J, Nassif PS. The more the merrier? Should antibiotics be used for rhinoplasty and septorhinoplasty – a review. Plast Reconstr Surg Glob Open 2018;6(10):e1972.

Management of Surgical Scars

Grace Lee Peng, MD[a],*, Julia L. Kerolus, MD[b]

KEYWORDS

- Hypertrophic scars • Keloids • Scar revision • Scars • Incisions • Wound healing
- Depressed scars • Microneedling

KEY POINTS

- Meticulous presurgical incision planning and wound closure are the first steps to avoiding the development of unsightly scars.
- Postoperative care of incisions includes maintaining a clean, moist environment to prevent inflammation and infection.
- Depressed scars can be treated with resurfacing, fillers, and scar revision.
- Hypertrophic scars and keloids are managed with a combination of various modalities including excision, radiation therapy, and intralesional injection of steroids, 5-fluorouracil, and botulinum toxin A.

INTRODUCTION

Surgical incisions will always result in a scar. What is important, however, is the final result of the scar after maturation. The goal is to have a scar that is minimally perceptible, with appropriate color match to the surrounding skin and be neither raised nor inverted. To ensure the best possible scar outcome, preoperative incision planning, wound tension during closure, and postsurgical management are all critical. Appropriate patient counseling and assessment of expectations is also important because patients often believe that a scar can be "removed."

Wound healing is a series of events starting from initial surgical incision that includes inflammation, proliferation, and remodeling.[1] It takes a year for the appearance of the scar to mature and even longer for the full strength of the scar to finalize. Initial inflammation after injury leads to chemotaxis of inflammatory cells and neovascularization, which in turn stimulates fibroblast proliferation. This leads to collagen production, and it is these events that can lead to either wound dehiscence or hypertrophy of scars.

PATIENT-RELATED FACTORS THAT AFFECT SCAR FORMATION

There are various patient-related factors that affect scar formation. Skin texture and color often predispose patients to different healing patterns. Thicker and more sebaceous skin often has more swelling after a surgical procedure. This swelling can lead to a longer healing time even after the sutures have been removed, because the edema even between where the sutures were placed may take longer to resolve. Similarly, even within an individual, the areas of thinner skin often heal much quicker and with less swelling. In general, African American and Asian patients are much more likely to have hypertrophic scarring and keloid formation in comparison with Caucasian patients.[2] With regard to hyperpigmentation, with

No financial disclosures.

[a] Facial Plastic and Reconstructive Surgery, 120 South Spalding Drive, Suite 301, Beverly Hills, CA 90212, USA;
[b] Department of Otolaryngology–Head and Neck Surgery, Division of Facial Plastic and Reconstructive Surgery, University of Illinois at Chicago-College of Medicine, 1855 West Taylor Street, Suite 2.42 (MC 648), Chicago, IL 60612, USA
* Corresponding author.
E-mail address: drpeng@graceleepengmd.com

Facial Plast Surg Clin N Am 27 (2019) 513–517
https://doi.org/10.1016/j.fsc.2019.07.013

all Fitzpatrick levels IV and higher there is a higher incidence of hyperpigmentation during wound healing regardless of the meticulous nature of the incision closure.[3]

A detailed surgical history obtained during preoperative consultation can give information on the patient's previous healing patterns after surgery. This information can help when deciding which intraoperative and postoperative measures are most crucial. In patients who have a history of hypertrophic scarring, care must be taken even with the sutures that are used to prevent any additional inflammation or irritation to the area of scar.

INTRAOPERATIVE MANAGEMENT
Incision Planning and Tissue Handling

Incisions should be planned so that they correspond to relaxed skin tension lines as often as possible.[3] Care should be taken to plan incisions at the junction of facial subunits to further decrease scar visibility after healing. In cases where incisions need to be made near hair-bearing areas, beveling the incision such that the hair can grow through the incision will allow the scar to be well hidden. Planning should also be done so that, for example in the case of facelifts or brow lifts, there is preservation of natural hair lines and hair-bearing areas.[4]

When handling the tissue, care must be taken not to traumatize the tissue by grabbing skin with improper forceps or with great force. One should always be gentle and, whenever possible, grabbing the deep dermal layer or subcutaneous layer is preferred over direct force on the skin surface itself.

Wound Closure

Skin tension pulls apart the edges of the wound and is often a reason for poor scar healing. The body counters tension by trying to hold the wound more tightly together, which leads to microscopic collagen deposition and increased scarring.[5] Thus, the tissue must be undermined. Placement of sutures in several layers whenever possible will help decrease the tension at the surface of the wound where the scar is visible. Maximal wound eversion is important to prevent the final scar from becoming depressed.

The sutures that are used also play a role for healing of surgical scars. In patients with more of a predisposition for aberrant wound healing, the use of less reactive and nonreactive sutures is preferred. Although Vicryl sutures are useful for their strength, duration, and ability to cause some scar tissue formation, some patients may

be more sensitive and develop an allergic reaction. Although this may not always lead to poor wound healing and visible scarring, there are ways to diminish this risk. Monocryl or polydioxanone sutures can be used for closure of deeper layers given their strength and lack of reactivity. In addition, for closure of the skin, nylon and Prolene sutures are less reactive than plain gut, fast gut, or chromic sutures. This aspect is important especially when dealing with patients who have more chance of hypertrophic scarring, prolonged erythema or hyperpigmentation, or postoperative swelling.

POSTOPERATIVE WOUND CARE
Immediate Postoperative Period

In the immediate postoperative period, the most important aspects to consider are to maintain moisture to the incision, prevent infection, and decrease inflammation.[3] All these facets need to be monitored while the tissue itself is healing the wound. Moisture can be maintained by an occlusive dressing or placement of ointment. Most commonly, antibiotic ointment is placed on the postoperative incision because it not only maintains the moisture but also helps to prevent infection. Prolonged use of antibiotic ointment is avoided because it may lead to skin irritation and inflammation. Keeping the incision clean and regularly removing any blood or crusting can further help to improve the skin healing.

One Week After Surgery

At 1 week, most if not all nonabsorbable sutures are removed. As the sutures are removed, tape can be placed on the incisions to decrease the tension.[6] At this time it is still very important to keep the wound moist. Although antibiotic ointment is no longer needed, especially for clean healing wounds without signs of infection, use of other occlusive ointments such as Aquaphor (Beiersdorf, Wilton, CT) can enhance wound healing.

Postoperative Care in the First Few Months

Topical treatments
By the second week, all the sutures should be removed if they have not already been removed. At this time, many clinicians will discuss the importance of using silicone sheets and gels to help in prevention of hypertrophic scarring.[7] The use of silicone gels and sheets appears to increase hydration to the stratum corneum, leading to improved wound healing.[8]

During this time, scars that will become hypertrophic may show signs early on. It is important to educate patients on the possibility that the appearance of the scar may change, and it is equally important to closely follow the healing of the scar. If the scar appears to be increasing in size or turning red and raised, the patient should be examined.

The use of intralesional injections with steroids or 5-fluorouracil (5-FU) can be used to decrease swelling and is discussed later in the section on treatment of hypertrophic scars and keloids.

Dermabrasion

The goal of dermabrasion is to even and blend the skin level in the raised area of scar; this can be achieved using diamond burrs, wire brushes, or sandpaper. The aim is to injure the papillary dermis to allow re-epithelialization and new collagen formation while preserving the deeper layers of skin. Any injury deeper than the papillary dermis, such as to the reticular dermis or below, leads to a greatly increased risk of scarring. Dermabrasion can be performed, with local anesthesia or topical numbing cream for comfort.

Constant reminders to the patient to decease direct sun exposure should be made. The patient should also be very diligent about sun protection in general to diminish the chance of increased inflammation or hyperpigmentation of the wound.[9]

VARIOUS TYPES OF SCARS AND THEIR MANAGEMENT
Depressed Scars

Depressed scars can often be prevented with careful and maximal eversion of every tissue layer during wound closure. When a depressed scar nevertheless appears, there is an indentation relative to the surrounding tissue. There are several ways to approach a depressed scar, such as resurfacing, filling the indentation, or performing a scar revision.

Microneedling

A depressed or inverted scar can be resurfaced by microneedling with platelet-rich plasma or hyaluronic acid. Microneedling, also known as collagen induction therapy, is a procedure whereby multiple small oscillating needles create damage to the area of the depressed scar. The body's response is to deposit collagen where the small punctures are created, hence increasing volume in the area of the depression. When paired with platelet-rich plasma, naturally occurring growth factors can further stimulate collagen production.[10] When the patient does not desire or is unable to use platelet-rich plasma, hyaluronic acid can be paired with microneedling.

Fillers

Depressed scars can also be filled in with either autologous grafts such as fat, collagen, or synthetic materials.[11,12] Some fillers can be permanent, but most lack permanence and thus over time may need reinjection. Subcision of a scar, depending on the location and length, may be helpful before filler placement to release any fibrous connections between the superficial scar and deep tissue. This approach allows for more effective filling of the area.

Scar revision

The other definitive treatment of depressed scars is scar revision and excision of the area of the scar. The goal is then to redo the closure such that with proper undermining and eversion of layers, the new scar will heal without an indentation. This method is the gold standard for repairing a depressed scar, although it usually cannot be done immediately after the initial procedure. Moreover, patients must be informed that the timeline for wound healing and all the precautions start anew with a scar revision.

Hypertrophic Scars and Keloids

Hypertrophic scars and keloids are due to abnormalities in the wound-healing process that lead to excess fibroproliferation as well as disorganized collagen deposition.[13,14] This process occurs more frequently in darker-skinned patients and can recur even after treatment. Whereas hypertrophic scars stay within the realm of the original incision and injury, a keloid actually extends beyond those original boundaries.[3,13]

Hypertrophic scars often appear reddish in color and can start growing as early as 3 months after the incision or injury.[15] Keloids may develop several months to even years later. Patients with a personal or family history of keloids should be followed closely for their incisions. Despite similar pathophysiology between hypertrophic scars and keloids, keloids have much lower rates of improvement when treated and a high recurrence rate after treatment.

Injections

Steroid injections can be used to manage or prevent hypertrophic scars and keloids. Corticosteroids can also decrease swelling, allowing for quicker wound healing. This injection is typically intradermal or transdermal, taking care not to inject any deeper to avoid causing tissue atrophy. There are many dilutions of triamcinolone that range from 5 mg/mL to 40 mg/mL. The strength used will depend on whether the goal is just to decrease swelling or to soften a hypertrophic scar or keloid.[16] Intralesional injections can inhibit collagen synthesis and increase degradation.[17,18] These injections can be repeated monthly.

5-FU injections have also been used in the treatment of keloids and hypertrophic scars. This approach can be taken even initially for swelling after surgery because the antimetabolite can prevent scar hypertrophy as well as decrease the size of some keloids.[3] 5-FU targets rapidly proliferating fibroblasts, which in turn lead to a decrease in collagen production and the formation of scar tissue.[19,20]

Recent studies have shown the benefit of intralesional injection of botulinum toxin type A in the treatment of keloids and hypertrophic scars.[21,22] The mechanism by which botulinum toxin A acts to prevent and treat hypertrophic scars is still unclear. Several theories have evolved from animal experiments. The theory is that botulinum toxin A decreases wound tension by paralysis of muscles and wound edges, downregulates fibroblast gene expression, and leads to thinning of collagen fibers.[23,24] This modality can be used alone or in conjunction with the aforementioned therapies. The risks associated with intralesional steroid injection, including skin atrophy, hypopigmentation, and telangiectasia formation, are nearly absent when botulinum toxin type A is injected alone. The amount injected varies among practitioners, types of scar, and purpose of injection (either preventing or treating scars). The dose range is from 2.5 to 100 units/cm^3.[22]

Radiotherapy
Low-dose fractionated radiotherapy after surgical excision of a keloid can be efficacious and safe.[8] Many times radiotherapy is avoided or used as a last resort owing to the small risk of malignancy. However, to date there have been no cases of malignancy reported after this use.

Pressure therapy
Pressure therapy can help both hypertrophic scars and keloids. After the wound has healed, physical pressure leads to a hypoxic environment and suppresses collagen production.[25] The recommended pressure exceeds 24 mm Hg for at least 30 min for upward of 12 months.[25,26] Although there have been some advances to make the pressure dressings easier to use and less burdensome, compliance has always been somewhat low because of the inconvenience and discomfort. Magnetic pressure earrings may be able to help keloids on the ear and earlobe if they are small and can be applied after large keloids are debulked. Keloids always run the risk of recurrence even after treatment has been completed.

Scar revision
When hypertrophic scars and keloids are nonresponsive to injections, they can be revised through excision scar revision. Using a Z-plasty or a W-plasty can help change the tension lines to alleviate any predisposition toward scar hypertrophy. Keloids have a high rate of recurrence despite surgical excision, and consequently need to be carefully monitored.

Hypopigmented Scars

Hypopigmented scars, or scars that are lacking in color, become noticeable because of a usually white and shiny appearance compared with the surrounding tissue. Hypopigmented scars can be covered with cosmetics which, although they may not permanently alter the scar, can have good results with easy achievability. If the patient desires a permanent solution, skin tattooing can produce good color-matching results.

Hyperpigmented Scars

Hyperpigmented scars can be of various colorations depending on the patient's native skin color and texture. Although hyperpigmentation is most often transient, long-term hyperpigmentation can draw more attention to the postsurgical scar. Much of hyperpigmentation is patient specific, but it can be influenced by external factors such as sun exposure after surgery.[9] UV light affects melanocyte proliferation and melanin deposition, leading to color change in the scar. Hence, avoidance of direct sunlight as well as good sun protection in the weeks to months immediately following the healing of a surgical scar leads to a decreased chance of hyperpigmentation.

Laser treatment
Traditionally, using pigment-specific lasers such as pulsed dye, potassium titanyl phosphate, or Nd:YAG lasers have had reasonable success.[5] However, microneedling or collagen induction therapy with platelet-rich plasma has also been known to show improvement in decreasing the pigmentation of scars. Topical remedies such as hydroquinone can also be used to lighten scars.

SUMMARY

Scarring is a significant source of morbidity for patients. Clinical management of postoperative scars begins preoperatively with through workup of each patient and understanding each individual's predisposition to poor scarring. The management and monitoring of surgical scars should continue for a year after surgery because the wound and incision can continue to change as it heals.

Postoperative visits should always be used to educate patients about scar care as well as to screen for any hypertrophy or hyperpigmentation.

Patients who are prone to hypertrophic scarring should be treated aggressively with injections of 5-FU, steroids, and botulinum toxin A. Careful identification of early development of hypertrophic scarring or keloid formation should be made and followed for an extended period of time.

As we continue to gain better understanding of wound healing, there are several options to improve postsurgical scars. However, there is no guarantee with any modality, either during or after surgery, for complete prevention of aberrant scar formation.

REFERENCES

1. Marshall CD, Hsu MS, Leavitt T, et al. Cutaneous scarring: basic science, current treatments, and future directions. Adv Wound Care (New Rochelle) 2018;7(2):29–45.
2. Gauglitz GG, Korting HC, Pavicic T, et al. Hypertrophic scarring and keloids: pathomechanisms and current and emerging treatment strategies. Mol Med 2011;17:113–25.
3. Chen MA, Davidson TM. Scar management: prevention and treatment strategies. Curr Opin Otolaryngol Head Neck Surg 2005;13:242–7.
4. Kridel RW, Liu ES. Techniques for creating inconspicuous face-lift scars: avoiding visible incisions and loss of temporal hair. Arch Facial Plast Surg 2003;5:325–33.
5. Son D, Harijian A. Overview of surgical scar prevention and management. J Korean Med Sci 2014;29:751–7.
6. Atkinson JA, McKenna KT, Barnett AG, et al. A randomized controlled trial to determine the efficacy of paper tape in preventing hypertrophic scar formation in surgical incisions that traverse Langer's skin tension lines. Plast Reconstr Surg 2005;116:1648–56.
7. Suetak T, Sasai S, Zhen YX, et al. Effects of silicone gel sheet on the stratum corneum hydration. Br J Plast Surg 2000;53:503–7.
8. Malaker K, Vijayraghavan K, Hodson I, et al. Retrospective analysis of treatment of unresectable keloid with primary radiation over 25 years. Clin Oncol 2004;16:290–8.
9. Chadwick S, Heath R, Shah M. Abnormal pigmentation with cutaneous scars: a complication of wound healing. Indian J Plast Surg 2012;45(2):403–11.
10. Ramut L, Hoeksema H, Pirayesh A, et al. Microneedling: where do we stand now? A systematic review of the literature. J Plast Reconstr Aesthet Surg 2011; 71:1–14.
11. De Benito J, Fernandex I, Nanda V. Treatment of depressed scars with a dissecting cannula and an autologous fat graft. Aesthetic Plast Surg 1999;23: 367–70.
12. Mak K, Toriumi D. Injectable filler materials for soft tissue augmentation. Otolaryngol Clin North Am 1994;27:211–22.
13. Thompson LDR. Skin keloid. Ear Nose Throat J 2004;83:519.
14. Torkian BA, Yeh AT, Engel R, et al. Modeling aberrant wound healing using tissue-engineered skin constructs and multiphoton microscopy. Arch Facial Plast Surg 2004;6:180–7.
15. Bran GM, Goessler UR, Hormann K, et al. Keloids: current concepts of pathogenesis (review). Int J Mol Med 2009;24:283–93.
16. Funcik T, Hochman M. The effect of intradermal corticosteroids on skin flap edema. Arch Otolaryngol Head Neck Surg 1995;121:654.
17. Tang YW. Intra and post operative steroid injections for keloids and hypertrophic scars. Br J Plast Surg 1992;45:371–3.
18. Rosen DJ, Patel MK, Freeman K, et al. A primary protocol for the management of ear keloids: results of excision combined with intraoperative and postoperative steroids injections. Plast Reconstr Surg 2007;120:1395–400.
19. Apikian M, Goodman G. Intralesional 5-fluorouracil in the treatment of keloid scars. Australas J Dermatol 2004;45:140.
20. LaRanger R, Karimpour-Fard A, Costa C, et al. Analysis of keloid response to 5-fluorouracil treatment and long-term prevention of keloid recurrence. Plast Reconstr Surg 2019;143(2):490–4.
21. Gamil HD, Khattab FM, El Fawal MN, et al. Comparison of intralesional triamcinolone acetonide, botulinum toxin type A, and their combination for the treatment of keloid lesions. J Dermatolog Treat 2019. [Epub ahead of print].
22. Kasyanju Carrero LM, Ma WW, Liu HF, et al. Botulinum toxin type A for the treatment and prevention of hypertrophic scars and keloids: updated review. J Cosmet Dermatol 2019;18(1):10–5.
23. Xiaoxue W, Xi C, Zhibo X. Effects of botulinum toxin type A on expression of genes in keloid fibroblasts. Aesthet Surg J 2014;34(1):154–9.
24. Zhibo X, Miaobo Z. Botulinum toxin type A affects cell cycle distribution of fibroblasts derived from hypertrophic scar. J Plast Reconstr Aesthet Surg 2008; 61(9):1128–9.
25. Niessen FB, Spauwen PH, Shalkwijk J, et al. On the nature of hypertrophic scars and keloids: a review. Plast Reconstr Surg 1999;104:1435–58.
26. Bouzari N, Davis SC, Nouri K. Laser treatment of keloids and hypertrophic scars. Int J Dermatol 2007; 46:80–8.

Common Complications in Rhytidectomy

Robert T. Cristel, MD[a],*, Leslie E. Irvine, MD[b]

KEYWORDS

• Facelift • Rhytidectomy • Complications • Avoidance

KEY POINTS

• The preoperative assessment is fundamental to predict, reduce, and avoid complications in rhytidectomy.
• Realistic expectations should be agreed on to avoid unexpected patient dissatisfaction.
• Hematoma is the most common immediate complication occurring within 24 hours.
• Facial nerve injury is a rare complication, with most being temporary, and should not dissuade surgeons from performing deeper dissections.
• Appropriate and timely management is crucial in minimizing poor outcomes from complications.

INTRODUCTION

Rhytidectomy remains one of the most popular surgical cosmetic procedures performed, as reported by the American Society for Aesthetic Plastic Surgery. In 2017, it ranked sixth among women, and fifth among men for surgical cosmetic treatments, with more than 80,000 performed.[1] With its continued popularity, it is prudent to recognize, prevent, and manage the well-known complications of facelift surgery.

Over the past century, new techniques have emerged to improve the aesthetic result advancing from skin-only facelift to superficial musculo-aponeurotic system (SMAS) manipulation techniques including SMAS plication, SMASectomy, deep plane, and others with varying degrees of SMAS dissection. Despite these new techniques, common complications remain, including hematomas, nerve injuries, skin necrosis, poor scars, and unsatisfactory cosmetic result. Fundamentally, the facelift surgeon should understand these common complications and learn to prevent, recognize early, and appropriately treat them

when present. This begins with the preoperative assessment.

PREOPERATIVE ASSESSMENT

The first encounter with a patient interested in rhytidectomy sets the framework for the operative plan and expected results. It is essential to have a thorough understanding of the patient's desires and motivations for surgery. Unrealistic expectations must be addressed and corrected preoperatively to avoid patient dissatisfaction following the procedure.

A complete history and physical examination provide important information about the patient's overall health and anticipates potential complications following the facelift. A history should include questioning of bleeding disorders, easy bruising, hypertension, anticoagulant use, cigarette smoking, diabetes, prescription and over-the-counter medications, herbal supplements, prior cosmetic procedures to the face and neck, and poor scarring or keloids. Further evaluation of cardiac, lung, or other major organ dysfunction should be

Disclosure Statement: The authors have no disclosures.
[a] Division of Facial Plastic and Reconstructive Surgery, Department of Otolaryngology–Head and Neck Surgery, University of Illinois at Chicago, 1855 West Taylor, Suite 2.42, Chicago, IL 60612, USA; [b] Santa Barbara Plastic Surgery Center, 222 West Pueblo Street, Suite A, Santa Barbara, CA 93105, USA
* Corresponding author.
E-mail address: rcrist3@uic.edu

Facial Plast Surg Clin N Am 27 (2019) 519–527
https://doi.org/10.1016/j.fsc.2019.07.008
1064-7406/19/© 2019 Elsevier Inc. All rights reserved.

addressed in the preoperative setting. Of increasing importance over the past several years, a history of neuromuscular blockade, filler injections, or other nonsurgical cosmetic treatments to the face and neck should be reviewed, as these can significantly impact the overall effect of the facelift procedure.

The physical examination should note the patient's desired areas for improvement and begin to plan a surgical technique tailored to the patient. Some signs of facial aging to assess include skin tone/laxity, rhytids, jowling, deepened nasolabial folds, prior scarring, prior filler placement, facial fat pads, jaw line, pre- and post-platysmal submental adiposity, and platysmal banding. The position of the hyoid can be used to discuss the best possible outcomes, with a high and posterior hyoid position being the most favorable to obtain an acute cervicomental angle.[2]

Two commonly overlooked areas are ptotic submandibular glands and prominent digastric muscles.[3] These can become more pronounced following submental liposuction. Removal of the submandibular glands adds increased risk of facial, lingual, and hypoglossal nerve injury and increased hematoma risk from facial and lingual artery bleeding.[3] The digastric muscles can be safely reduced or partially removed using a suction bovie. Assessment of temporal and mastoid hairlines is also necessary to plan for incision placement. Patients, particularly men, who have preoperative hair loss should be identified, and prevention of further loss is of great importance for patient satisfaction.

Any facial nerve irregularities should be noted before the procedure. A history of Bell palsy should be discussed. If facial asymmetry is noted, this should be documented and reviewed with the patient to prevent confusion in the postoperative period (**Fig. 1**).

Interestingly, the age of the patient can influence the perceived results and satisfaction of facelift

surgery. The ideal age has been found to be 50 or younger based on patient satisfaction studies.[2] Patients may tend to wait until more significant signs of aging are present, but patients older than 50 report lower satisfaction and decreased long-term outcomes as well.[2] Patients presenting at a slightly younger age also have the option of newer techniques, such as the short scar facelift when the signs of aging may not be as severe. As aging continues, the short scar technique may not be as effective for achieving optimum results, particularly in the neck.

LOCAL ANESTHETIC

Whether performed under local or general anesthesia, local anesthetic with epinephrine is near universally used. Proper dosage should be strictly accounted for, as a significant amount may be required with extensive dissections. Many surgeons also mix lidocaine with bupivacaine, among other local anesthetics, and the different concentrations must be accounted for to avoid complications. If under general anesthesia, intravenous lidocaine may also be used before intubation and should be calculated into the maximum dosing.[4]

Local anesthetic toxicity presents with central nervous system findings before cardiovascular effects. Neurologic effects include lightheadedness, dizziness, perioral numbness, tremors, and seizures.[5] However, these may not be appreciated if under general anesthesia. Cardiovascular collapse, such as hypotension and arrhythmias are further signs of local anesthetic toxicity and must be treated immediately in coordination with the anesthesia team.

COMPLICATIONS

Although some of the common complications in rhytidectomy may initially seem devastating to both patient and surgeon, the long-term sequelae are often minimal with appropriate follow-up care. A thorough understanding of facelift complications and their timing will provide a framework for avoidance and management.

HEMATOMA

Hematomas are the most common postoperative complication in rhytidectomy and typically develop within the first 24 hours (**Fig. 2**). The incidence requiring surgical intervention ranges from 1% to 15%; however, is more commonly noted in the 1% to 5% range.[4,5] The use of ice, pressure dressing, and adequate hemostasis intraoperatively are the universal techniques in hematoma

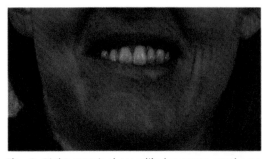

Fig. 1. Right marginal mandibular nerve weakness. This is important to document during the preoperative examination.

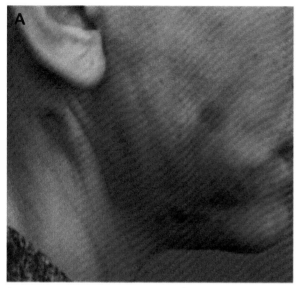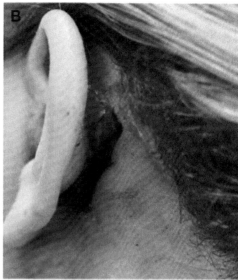

Fig. 2. Hematoma sequelae. (*A*) Prolonged bruising 16 days after facelift complicated by hematoma requiring evacuation in the operating room. (*B*) Postauricular necrosis and scar erythema apparent on postoperative day 16.

prevention. Suction drains are commonly used but have not been definitively shown to reduce hematoma risk.[6]

Male gender is an independent risk factor representing the increased incidences. This can be attributed to a higher number of perfused facial microvessels in male skin, particularly underlying the facial hair distribution and sebaceous glands.[4,7]

An expanding hematoma presents with sudden, acute pain with swelling, ecchymosis, tense skin, trismus, anxiety, and potential airway compromise if located in the neck. An expanding hematoma necessitates and urgent wound exploration and control of bleeding to prevent compromise to the overlying skin. If controlled quickly, the final aesthetic result is usually not compromised.[3] If left untreated, skin necrosis may develop, leading to worse wound healing and poor scarring.

There are many patient factors to consider in preventing hematoma formation. Preoperatively, patients should be instructed to avoid aspirin, nonsteroidal anti-inflammatory drugs, and herbal supplements that may increase bleeding risk for 2 weeks before surgery. Common herbal supplements to observe for include Ginkgo biloba, ginseng, garlic, St. John's wort, vitamin E, kava, and licorice.[3] Because of the increased prevalence of herbal supplements without Food and Drug Administration regulations, it is best to have patients stop all herbal supplements 2 weeks before surgery to avoid any confusion or potential unknown side effects.

If a patient requires anticoagulation, such as warfarin, rivaroxaban, heparin, or clopidogrel, communication with the primary care provider regarding stopping and restarting their use is essential. As facelift is an elective procedure, it is important to realize that underlying medical problems may eliminate a patient's candidacy for surgery.

Hypertension is another known and controllable risk factor for hematoma. Particularly in known hypertensive patients, adequate preoperative control is key; however, postoperative spikes are often the culprit, even in nonhypertensive patients. The threshold systolic pressure is typically reported to be >150 mm Hg.[3,5] Close communication intraoperatively with the anesthesia team is another critical factor. On awakening, if under general anesthesia, a smooth wake up and extubation can decrease the amount of retching, Valsalva, and blood pressure spikes. Ensuring appropriate pain and nausea control, particularly within the first 24 hours, can help prevent hematoma formation. Consideration of short-term blood pressure control in previously nondiagnosed hypertensive patients is warranted, although no formal guidelines exist.

Hypotensive anesthesia may contribute to increased hematoma risk by keeping blood pressure unnaturally low and masking vessels that may bleed once normal blood pressure is restored when the patient is awake.[8]

Tissue sealants have remained controversial despite their growth in popularity among facial plastic surgeons. A recent meta-analysis demonstrated a significant reduction of hematoma rates using tissue sealants with a relative risk of 0.37.[9] Although hematoma rates decreased, seroma rates remained unchanged and drain usage was not decreased with tissue sealants.

Facelift approach has limited effect on hematoma rates. A meta-analysis showed that a deep plane dissection had increased hematoma risk requiring surgical revision compared with SMAS plication alone.[10] This study had a relatively low odds ratio of 1.68, so the investigators concluded that there is no clinical significance and avoidance of deep plane dissections is not warranted. In other instances, particularly smokers, a deep plane technique can lower hematoma rates.[10] A deeper plane limits the dissection of the underlying subdermal plexus. This maneuver allows for increased blood supply and venous drainage to the skin flap, preventing skin necrosis, and possibly lowering hematoma rates.[10]

FACIAL NERVE INJURY

Facial nerve injury is the most dreaded complication of facelift surgery. In a review of medical malpractice cases related to rhytidectomy, damage to the facial nerve and intraoperative negligence were the top 2 allegations most likely to lead to payment to plaintiffs.[11] Nerve injury has been reported to occur in 0.5% to 2.5% of cases with permanent nerve injury at 0.1%.[3,5] Despite the low occurrences, the theoretic risk with deeper and more extensive dissection remains, and cautions some surgeons away from these techniques.

The frontal and marginal mandibular branches are the most affected due to the limited interconnections compared with the other branches of the facial nerve. Adequate knowledge of facial nerve anatomy is essential with SMAS manipulation. The frontal branch runs just deep to the SMAS over the zygomatic arch; therefore, skin dissection should occur in a subcutaneous plane to avoid injury.[12–14] The marginal mandibular nerve is most commonly affected along the caudal border of the mandible, where it may run above or below the mandible. There is potential for injury even during liposuction of the submental region if the platysma is tented by retraction and the cannula proceeds deep to the platysma muscle.[5,14]

If the facial nerve is clearly transected proximal to a vertical line along the lateral canthus, then primary repair should be performed.[15] This would be a very rare event. The more common scenario involves temporary facial weakness due to stretching, heat injury, or edema. Cautery should be used judiciously, and only bipolar cautery should be used, near the facial nerve to reduce neuropraxia.

Postoperatively, local anesthesia can cause asymmetry, and this may take several hours to wear off. If nerve injury has caused asymmetry and it is particularly bothersome to the patient, the use of neuromodulators such as Botox can be used on the nonaffected side to achieve better symmetry. As most facial nerve injuries are temporary, this may require only 1 to 2 treatments of neurotoxin before full nerve function returns. Patient education and reassurance are necessary, as formal exploration for nerve injury is not typically required.

GREAT AURICULAR NERVE INJURY

The great auricular nerve is much more commonly injured during facelift surgery, with an incidence up to 7%.[5] Although this is a sensory nerve, it can still create significant discomfort for patients, with paresthesia and even pain in the preauricular region and lower portion of the ear. The great auricular nerve runs deep to sternocleidomastoid (SCM) fascia and originates from the Erb point approximately 6.5 cm inferior to the external acoustic meatus, commonly along the posterior border of the SCM.

The posterior neck flap dissection must be done very superficially to avoid exposing the fascia over the SCM and prevent nerve injury. If injury occurs and is readily available for repair, it should be repaired to prevent paresthesia. If not transected, sensation generally returns within a few months, or at least a level that is insignificant to the patient. If permanent numbness remains over a significant portion of the ear, patients must be instructed to use proper ear protection in cold weather to prevent the risk of frostbite.

Although numbness is the primary complaint following great auricular nerve injury, pain also may develop. Neuromas following transection have been reported to cause intractable pain.[15] Trials of gabapentin or low-dose tricyclic antidepressants (TCAs) are beneficial for chronic neuropathic pain in this region with improvement noted in most patients at 12 months. However, removal of a neuroma may remain necessary in some cases, which provides more definitive relief.[16]

OTHER NERVE INJURIES

Although the facial nerve and great auricular nerve are the most commonly discussed nerve injuries, several other nerves remain at risk during rhytidectomy. The lesser occipital nerve, also located along the posterior border of the SCM, is at risk in a dissection similar to the great auricular nerve. This injury would create numbness and possible paresthesia to the posterior ear.

Even more posteriorly, the spinal accessory nerve can be injured with deep dissection. The spinal accessory nerve is located within 2 cm of the Erb point along the posterior SCM, either superior or inferior. Shoulder weakness, asymmetry, or winged scapula may occur as a result of injury, potentially necessitating physical therapy while awaiting for nerve function to return.[3,4] If paresthesias are present, similar medication trial with gabapentin or low-dose TCAs may be warranted. Understanding of anatomy will help prevent these complications.

SKIN FLAP NECROSIS

Skin flap necrosis can be particularly bothersome and concerning to patients because of the obvious discoloration and poor wound healing that occurs (see Fig. 2). However, local therapy and watchful waiting are the cornerstones for this complication. Necrosis is caused by vascular congestion and/or arterial compromise from edema, hematoma, or damage to the subdermal plexus during flap dissection.[3] Limited bipolar cautery is used to prevent disruption of blood supply to the overlying skin flap.

Smoking increases the risk of skin flap necrosis 12- to 20-fold.[5,17] Smoking creates both acute vasoconstriction and long-term changes to the microvasculature, including obliterative endarteritis. This increases the likelihood of thrombogenesis, poor wound healing, and tissue hypoxia.[18] Patients should be warned preoperatively about this increased risk. Ideally, patients should refrain from smoking 4 weeks before and 4 weeks after surgery. This remains a very difficult compromise for many. A urinary screen for cotinine, a urinary metabolite for nicotine, is available and detects smoking for up to 4 days if poor compliance is suspected.[16,17]

If skin flap necrosis occurs, it is typically in the postauricular or preauricular regions, as these are the regions of most tension on closure. A properly designed incision and thorough closure with deep sutures to relieve tension is important for prevention of necrosis. If severe, it can be beneficial to release any sutures that are causing tension to allow for increased vascularity to the area. Local wound care with antibiotic ointment is typically sufficient for management. An eschar may develop and provides a local pressure dressing, therefore removal is not usually performed. Topical nitroglycerin is also commonly used in these areas, although evidence is lacking in its benefit.[3,15]

Close patient follow-up is recommended, as the area of necrosis can become rather unsightly. Reassurance is essential, as long-term healing is generally cosmetically favorable. There are many nonsurgical treatment options for scars that are available once appropriate healing time has been allowed. These will be reviewed in a subsequent article. (see article "Management of Surgical Scars" by Grace Lee Peng and Julia Kerolus in this issue.)

SCARRING

Incision planning is key to scar outcomes. Poor scarring is one of the most important aspects of patient satisfaction after facelift surgery. The incision must be planned to both hide the scar and to avoid alterations of the hairline. Incisions in non–hair-bearing skin should be placed within natural contours of the preauricular and postauricular regions. In men, the preauricular incision is classically pretragal to prevent facial hair from being pulled into the tragal cartilage.[5] In women the incision is retrotragal for better camouflage.

In hair-bearing areas, the incision should be beveled parallel to hair follicles to avoid alopecia. In bald men, a broken line incision instead of a linear incision in the temporal and occipital areas can camouflage postoperative scars (Fig. 3). To minimize hypertrophic scarring, a detailed, multilayered closure must be performed to reduce tension and prevent widening of the incision.

Hypo/hyperpigmentation also may occur. Standard sun protection is recommended to avoid worsening scar discoloration. If unfavorable scarring occurs, intralesional steroid and 5-fluorouracil injections, silicone sheeting, laser treatments, medical tattooing for hypopigmentation, among other advancements in scar revision, are available for treatment.[3,15] These will be reviewed in a separate article. (see article "Management of Surgical Scars" by Grace Lee Peng and Julia Kerolus in this issue.)

EAR DEFORMITY

Tragal displacement and earlobe deformity are the 2 most common auricular complications. Anterior displacement of the tragus can occur, creating an unnatural appearance. Proper skin redraping, a tension-free closure, and placing a tacking stitch through the skin into the tragal perichondrium to re-create the pretragal notch can prevent this complication. If persistent deformity remains, correction should be completed at least 6 months and ideally 12 months postoperatively to allow for full contracture to occur before revision.

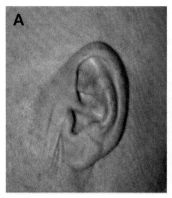 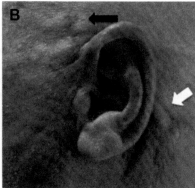 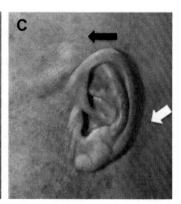

Fig. 3. (*A*) Before, (*B*) 1 month after, and (*C*) 1 year after facelift in a bald patient who had a broken line incision in the temporal area (*black arrows*) and a linear closure in the occipital area (*white arrows*).

Pixie ear can be an even more obvious deformity (**Fig. 4**). This occurs when the earlobe is pulled inferiorly and the sulcus between the earlobe and cheek is obliterated, creating the appearance of the earlobe inserting directly into the cheek. Prevention is key for pixie ear deformity. Leaving a small amount of redundant skin beneath the earlobe to allow for scar contracture prevents the inferior displacement of the earlobe.[3,5] If deformity of the earlobe persists, excision of the scar with V-Y advancement of the earlobe can allow for correction as early as 6 months postoperatively.[3]

SEROMA

Seromas typically present approximately 2 to 7 days postoperatively and are most commonly postauricular or infra-auricular. These may be treated with percutaneous needle aspiration and pressure dressing. Removal of fluid restores blood supply to the skin flap and reduces risk of infection. Although tissue sealants have been shown to reduce hematoma formation and output from suction drains, they have not been shown to reduce the incidence of seromas.[9] The decreased serous fluid in the wound though, can have potential benefits of decreasing wound infections and healing time.[9]

PAROTID DUCT INJURY

Injuries to the parotid gland or ductal system remain rare, although are more common with deeper sub-SMAS dissections. If injury to the parenchyma occurs, cautery can be used to seal the injury, along with tight closure of the SMAS over the defect. There remains the possibility of sialocele development, which can be managed with serial aspirations, compression dressings,

and scopolamine patches.[19] Botulinum toxin also can be used for persistent sialoceles.[3,15]

Injury to the Stenson duct can occur along the anterior border of the masseter during sub-SMAS dissection. If an injury is noted, a catheter may be cannulated from the oral cavity retrograde into the proximal injured end. The duct can then be sutured and cannula removed in approximately 2 weeks as long as no evidence of sialocele remains.[3]

HAIR LOSS

Rates of alopecia are as high as 8%, although most hair loss is temporary with only 1% to 3% being permanent.[3] As with other complications, prevention is the primary technique to avoid complications. Hair loss is most commonly along the temporal hairline and can be from damage to the follicles during incision, electrocautery, excessive tension with closure, or hypertrophic scarring. Occipital hair loss is less frequent.

Patients with hair loss preoperatively are at increased risk for postoperative alopecia. Topical minoxidil has been shown to be effective in preventing the incidence of alopecia and increasing the recovery time if present.[3,4] Although alopecia can be bothersome, reassurance to the patient that it is most commonly temporary is important. A full 12 months should be allowed for recovery to occur before any further treatment options are pursued.

POOR AESTHETIC OUTCOMES

Unfortunately, despite proper technique and planning, poor aesthetic outcomes and patient dissatisfaction may occur. In the immediate postoperative period, there remains significant edema and ecchymosis that can distort the

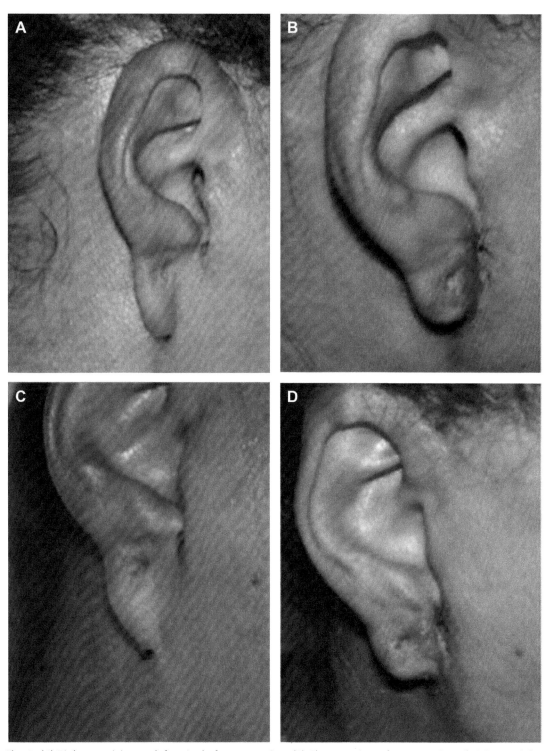

Fig. 4. (*A*) Right ear pixie ear deformity before correction. (*B*) Close up view after correction of pixie ear deformity with wide skin undermining and advancement flap. (*C*) Close up pixie ear deformity before correction. (*D*) After correction of pixie ear deformity with wide skin undermining and advancement flap.

final result. Time for healing must be allowed to gain a true sense of any poor results. Massage, head elevation, low-salt diet, ice packs, and incisional care are conservative measures in the early postoperative period to reduce edema.

During the initial history and physical examination, patients should be advised about possible persistent deformities following surgery, particularly in patients with low and anterior hyoids, ptotic submandibular glands, prominent digastric muscles, and microgenia. Although setting expectations will not dissipate all dissatisfaction, it helps create an open communication between patient and physician about expected results.

There may be persistent nasolabial folds, jowls, prejowl sulci, rhytids, and platysma bands, to name a few. Ptotic submandibular glands often become more prominent following submental liposuction, along with facelift, and patients should be warned about this possibility. Excessive submental liposuction can lead to a hollowed appearance of the upper neck known as cobra neck deformity. Improper platysmal plication worsens this appearance. This can be prevented with conservative fat excision. Severe deformities may be treated with autologous fat transfer after allowing 12 months of healing.[3]

There are many different facelift techniques including, but not limited to, SMAS plication, SMASectomy, SMAS flap, high lateral SMAS flap, deep plane, and composite.[20] There remains significant controversy and continuous discussions about which technique provides the best aesthetic result and long-term outcome. Because of difficulty in blinded prospective studies regarding rhytidectomy, true comparisons among aesthetic outcomes are difficult and sparse. The techniques used ultimately relies on individualized preoperative decision-making and the surgeon's experience and expertise. There is no consistent technique that has been shown to provide the most favorable aesthetic result with the best long-term outcomes.

As many small defects, such as skin nodules or puckering, can remain present for several months after facelift, more significant treatment options should wait a period of 12 months. If persistent deformities remain, these may be treated with autologous fat injections, injectable fillers, neuromodulators, CO_2 lasers, and other new emerging technologies in the field of nonsurgical facial rejuvenation.

Ecchymosis is a common finding and usually resolves within 2 to 3 weeks. Corticosteroids have not been found to have an effect on the amount of edema or ecchymosis.[17] Hyperbaric oxygen has been found to promote faster wound healing. There was no effect on skin necrosis, however, at postoperative day 7, and beyond there was reduced ecchymosis.[21] Hyperbaric oxygen therapy may be a good option for patients very concerned with shortening the recovery period, but this must be weighed with an estimated cost of $1100 for the full effect.[21]

INFECTION

Fortunately, infection following facelift is rare and reported to be less than 1%.[3] When recognized and treated promptly with antibiotic therapy, it will not have long-lasting cosmetic effects. If there is concern for chondritis, coverage for *Pseudomonas* is necessary, otherwise coverage for *Staphylococcus* and *Streptococcus* is sufficient.

DEEP VEIN THROMBOSIS

Although rare, deep vein thrombosis (DVT) and pulmonary embolism are potential devastating and life-threatening complications of facelift surgery. With a reported incidence of 0.1%, the risk remains low, but proactive measures always should be taken.[3,5] Intermittent compression stockings in local and general anesthesia cases always should be worn. Early mobilization is a universal standard that should be followed.

Chemical prophylaxis when performed under general anesthesia remains controversial, as studies have reported an increased incidence of hematoma (up to 16%) in patients receiving low molecular weight heparin for DVT prophylaxis.[22] The risks and benefits must be weighed for each individual patient based on past medical history, local or general anesthesia, and predicted operative time. Operative time of 5 hours or longer was associated with an increased risk of DVT.[3]

SUMMARY

Facelift complications are well known. Planning for ways to prevent their occurrence should occur in every preoperative patient assessment. The preoperative assessment is fundamental to predict, reduce, and avoid complications in rhytidectomy. Transparent communication and setting realistic expectations are critical to avoid unexpected patient dissatisfaction. A close patient-physician relationship can ameliorate detrimental outcomes and improve patient satisfaction.

Complications are often treated conservatively with close postoperative follow-up. Hematoma is the most common complication, typically occurring within 24 hours, and may require return to the operating room. The theoretic risk of facial nerve injury in deeper dissections continues to push surgeons toward other techniques, yet permanent damage is extremely rare. Although many facelift techniques exist, there is no universal standard for which provides the best outcomes with the lowest complication rates. Proper preoperative evaluation, surgical planning, and complication management are key to a successful rhytidectomy.

REFERENCES

1. Surgery, A.S.f.A.P.. Cosmetic surgery national data bank statistics. 2017. Available at: https://www.surgery.org/sites/default/files/ASAPS-Stats2017.pdf. Accessed March 26, 2019.
2. Marcus BC. Rhytidectomy: current concepts, controversies and the state of the art. Curr Opin Otolaryngol Head Neck Surg 2012;20(4):262–6.
3. Chaffoo RA. Complications in facelift surgery: avoidance and management. Facial Plast Surg Clin North Am 2013;21(4):551–8.
4. Moyer JS, Baker SR. Complications of rhytidectomy. Facial Plast Surg Clin North Am 2005;13(3):469–78.
5. Clevens RA. Avoiding patient dissatisfaction and complications in facelift surgery. Facial Plast Surg Clin North Am 2009;17(4):515–30, v.
6. Jones BM, Grover R, Hamilton S. The efficacy of surgical drainage in cervicofacial rhytidectomy: a prospective, randomized, controlled trial. Plast Reconstr Surg 2007;120(1):263–70.
7. Rohrich RJ, Stuzin JM, Ramanadham S, et al. The modern male rhytidectomy: lessons learned. Plast Reconstr Surg 2017;139(2):295–307.
8. Moris V, Bensa P, Gerenton B, et al. The cervicofacial lift under pure local anaesthesia diminishes the incidence of post-operative haematoma. J Plast Reconstr Aesthet Surg 2019;72(5):821–9.
9. Giordano S, Koskivuo I, Suominen E, et al. Tissue sealants may reduce haematoma and complications in face-lifts: a meta-analysis of comparative studies. J Plast Reconstr Aesthet Surg 2017;70(3):297–306.
10. Jacono AA, Sean Alemi A, Russell JL. A meta-analysis of complication rates among different SMAS facelift techniques. Aesthet Surg J 2019. [Epub ahead of print].
11. Kandinov A, Mutchnick S, Nangia V, et al. Analysis of factors associated with rhytidectomy malpractice litigation cases. JAMA Facial Plast Surg 2017;19(4):255–9.
12. Visconti G, Salgarello M. Anatomical considerations to prevent facial nerve injury: insights on frontal branch and cervicofacial trunk nerve anatomy in SMAS face lifts. Plast Reconstr Surg 2016;137(4):751e–2e.
13. Connell BF, Marten TJ. The trifurcated SMAS flap: three-part segmentation of the conventional flap for improved results in the midface, cheek, and neck. Aesthetic Plast Surg 1995;19(5):415–20.
14. Roostaeian J, Rohrich RJ, Stuzin JM. Anatomical considerations to prevent facial nerve injury. Plast Reconstr Surg 2015;135(5):1318–27.
15. Fedok FG. The avoidance and management of complications, and revision surgery of the lower face and neck. Clin Plast Surg 2018;45(4):623–34.
16. Chopra K, Kokosis G, Slavin B, et al. Painful complications after cosmetic surgery: management of peripheral nerve injury. Aesthet Surg J 2018. [Epub ahead of print].
17. Derby BM, Codner MA. Evidence-based medicine: face lift. Plast Reconstr Surg 2017;139(1):151e–67e.
18. Wan D, Small KH, Barton FE. Face lift. Plast Reconstr Surg 2015;136(5):676e–89e.
19. Lapid O, Kreiger Y, Sagi A. Transdermal scopolamine use for post-rhytidectomy sialocele. Aesthetic Plast Surg 2004;28(1):24–8.
20. Floyd EM, Sukato DC, Perkins SW. Advances in face-lift techniques, 2013-2018: a systematic review. JAMA Facial Plast Surg 2019;21(3):252–9.
21. Stong BC, Jacono AA. Effect of perioperative hyperbaric oxygen on bruising in face-lifts. Arch Facial Plast Surg 2010;12(5):356–8.
22. Guyuron B. An evidence-based approach to face lift. Plast Reconstr Surg 2010;126(6):2230–3.

Neck Deformities in Plastic Surgery

Neil A. Gordon, MD[a,b,*], Boris Paskhover, MD[c,d], Jacob I. Tower, MD[e],
Thomas Gerald O'Daniel, MD, FACS, EMBA[f,1]

KEYWORDS

- Neck lift • Complications • Platysma • Subplatysma surgery • Revision • Submandibular gland
- Digastric muscle • Deep central neck fat

KEY POINTS

- With respect to neck procedures, the major anatomic structure in the neck is the platysma muscle, which divides the neck into superficial and deep anatomic compartments.
- Although platysma and supraplatysma fat are the most commonly addressed structures in neck lift procedures, all anatomic structures can contribute to an unsatisfactory neck appearance and need to be accurately assessed and treated for optimal results.
- Complications in neck surgery can result from well-planned, well-designed, and well-executed procedures.
- Complications in appearance often occur because of imbalances in treatment between superficial and deep neck structures.
- Because of ease of access, overcorrection of the preplatsymal space is common, whereas difficulty of access leads to an undercorrection of the subplatysmal space.

INTRODUCTION

In discussing complications, their sequelae, and potential solutions in surgery of the neck, the initial treatment goals should first be defined. The appearance of the optimal neck was defined by Ellenbogen and Karlin[1] in a 1980 article in which they listed 5 visual criteria of an elegant neck contour. The components include smooth skin with the absence of redundancy, rhytids and horizontal crease, a well-defined jawline, and absence of platysmal bands. In addition, the structures of the deep central neck, including the subplatysmal fat, digastric muscles, submandibular glands, and perihyoid fascia, must also be appropriately addressed (**Fig. 1**).

Significant variations in native neck anatomy can make many of these criteria either simple or difficult to achieve. Surgical intervention in the neck can have 2 basic goals: to create a neck contour that is an improvement compared with the native anatomy, or, in facial rejuvenation, to restore the original anatomy that has been compromised by time. Surgical interventions can be isolated to the neck or, commonly in facial rejuvenation, combined with other facial plastic procedures.

Disclosure: The authors have no financial conflicts of interest to disclose.
[a] New England Surgical Center, The Retreat at Split Rock, 539 Danbury Road, Wilton, CT 06897, USA; [b] Head and Neck Aesthetic Surgery, Facial Plastic and Reconstructive Surgery, Department of Surgery, Section of Otolaryngology, Yale School of Medicine, New Haven, CT, USA; [c] Department of Otolaryngology–Head and Neck Surgery, Rutgers New Jersey Medical School, Newark, NJ, USA; [d] Facial Plastics and Reconstructive Surgery, St. Barnabas Medical Center, Robert Wood Johnson Barnabas Health, Livingston, NJ, USA; [e] Department of Surgery, Section of Otolaryngology, Yale School of Medicine, 800 Howard Avenue, 4th Floor YPB, New Haven, CT 06519, USA; [f] Department of Plastic Surgery, University of Louisville, 132 Chenoweth Lane, Louisville, KY 40207, USA
[1] Senior author.
* Corresponding author. New England Surgical Center, The Retreat at Split Rock, 539 Danbury Road, Wilton, CT.
E-mail address: ngordon@splitrocksurgical.com

Facial Plast Surg Clin N Am 27 (2019) 529–555
https://doi.org/10.1016/j.fsc.2019.07.009

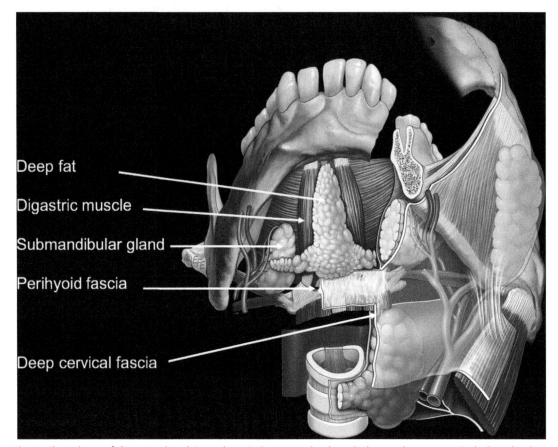

Deep fat

Digastric muscle

Submandibular gland

Perihyoid fascia

Deep cervical fascia

Fig. 1. The volume of the central neck is made up in large part by the subplatysmal structures, including the deep fat, digastric muscles, and submandibular glands. In addition, the perihyoid fascia can contribute to an obtuse cervicomental angle. The deep neck structures are beneath the deep cervical fascia, which has implications for bleeding when managing the deep neck structures. Procedure performed by T. Gerald O'Daniel, MD, FACS. (*Courtesy of* T. Gerald O'Daniel, MD, FACS, O'Daniel Plastic Surgery Studios, Louisville, KY.)

As in any surgery, a detailed understanding of the anatomy of the neck is paramount to effectively perform comprehensive neck surgery and to understand the occurrence of certain complications and their potential remedies.[2]

The major anatomic structure in the neck is the platysma muscle. From the Greek word for plate, this quadrangular sheet of muscle is invested within the superficial cervical fascia of the head and neck, extending from the fascia of the pectoralis major inferiorly to the body of the mandible and extending cephalad by incorporating into the superficial musculoaponeurotic system (SMAS) of the midface. As the underbelly of the superficial soft tissue envelope of the midface and neck, and the boundary between superficial soft tissue and deeper, structural aspects of the face and neck, the platysma is affected by aging changes unlike any other muscle.

Using the platysma muscle as a divide, complications can be segregated because of either commission or omission of structures superficial or deep to this muscle. Conceptually, complications in appearance often occur because of imbalances between the superficial neck soft tissue and the deep neck structures, with either being undertreated/overtreated with respect to the corresponding region. This situation often occurs because of the ease, or difficulty, of access of certain anatomic regions of the neck. Accordingly, the overcorrection of the preplatysmal space and undercorrection of subplatysma space tend to be common.

Complications can arise from any well-designed and well-executed procedure, such as hematoma/seroma, as well as in poorly designed and performed procedures, such as poor incisions and excessive tension. Similar-appearing complications can have multiple different causes, such as neck contour deformities. Although emphasis in neck complication discussions is often placed on surgical issues accompanying face/neck lift surgery and primary neck liposuction, a new focus needs to be placed on advent of the minimally invasive techniques. Although termed nonsurgical, significant short-term complications have been defined with these techniques, and long-term issues are only beginning to be seen.

TREATMENT OPTIONS

There are many described neck lift operations that attempt to create the optimal neck contour. These procedures can be described as a lateral approach, with or without an open central neck procedure, or closed neck procedures.

Various lateral approach procedures manage the jawline and neck by addressing soft tissue redundancy associated with aging via a facelift incision through repositioning and fixation of the SMAS and/or the lateral platysma,[3,4] and can include indirect treatment of the central platysma from laterally based platysma manipulation and fixation.[5,6] Often suction-assisted liposuction is combined with the lateral approach to reduce the supraplatysmal fat.

Because of limitations in results in the central neck from a lateral-only approach, open neck procedures, referring to the direct approach to the central neck with a submental incision, have been advocated by numerous investigators.[7–9] This approach to the central neck with a submental incision is used in isolation for neck lifting in young patients or combined with the lateral approach to achieve optimal neck contour by addressing both the soft tissue redundancy as well as the central neck structures both superficial (supraplatysmal fat and laxity of the platysma) and deep (subplatysmal fat, digastric muscles, submandibular glands, perihyoid fascia).

Closed neck procedures in the past have referred mainly to various forms of liposuction, but in the last decade there has been an expansion in the growth of nonsurgical and minimally invasive technologies designed to improve the appearance of the neck. These technologies include energy-based devices that attempt to tighten skin and reduce supraplatysmal fat and affect the platysma. In addition, cryotreatment devices and enzymatic agents have been approved for reduction of the supraplatysmal fat. With the increasing number of patients receiving these treatments clinicians are now being presented with complications that require surgical intervention to correct.[10]

COMPLICATIONS
Hematoma

Hematoma formation is the most common complication following rhytidectomy, and of particular relevance when rejuvenation procedures include neck lifting. Postoperative hematoma is reported to occur in up to 15% of rhytidectomy patients, and in one large analysis it was the cause of 62% of all rhytidectomy complications.[11]

Typically, expanding hematomas occur within the first 24 hours after surgery and require prompt evacuation, often in the operating room, to prevent sequelae. In contrast, minor hematomas may appear days or even weeks after surgery and can often be managed with simple bedside aspiration (**Fig. 2**). Hematomas require prompt attention to avoid delayed recovery, skin loss, potential

A

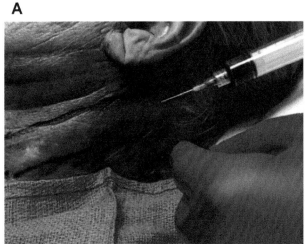

B

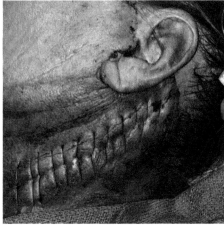

Fig. 2. (*A*) Patient 10 days after face and neck lift with a liquefied hematoma in the left lateral neck. Aspiration was performed to remove blood. (*B*) A hemostatic net was placed. A 5-0 nylon continuous running suture closed the skin against the deep tissues. Procedure performed by T. Gerald O'Daniel, MD, FACS. (*Courtesy of* T. Gerald O'Daniel, MD, FACS, O'Daniel Plastic Surgery Studios, Louisville, KY.)

airway compromise, and delayed issues related to pigmentary changes and contour deformities from the subcutaneous scarring.

The authors' approach to prevention of hematomas includes cessation of aspirin, nonsteroidal antiinflammatory drugs, and other platelet-inhibiting agents. Perioperative management includes hematoma prevention through hypotensive anesthesia technique. Although we prefer general anesthesia, the senior author (T.G.O'D.), has used an intravenous sedation method using dexmedetomidine (Precedex) as the primary sedative for the last 15 years.[12] What differentiates dexmedetomidine from narcotics and propofol is that it is able to achieve its effects without respiratory depression. It is an alpha agonist that is effective in controlling intraoperative blood pressure, with an optimal mean of 60 mm Hg, while potentiating the effect of narcotics and anxiolytic agents. The half-life of Precedex is 2 hours, which helps with blood pressure control at the conclusion of the surgery, when it is especially important.

In addition, some authors use suction drains and a pressure dressing. The pressure dressing is applied in the operating room and the submental portion is significantly loosened in the midline 1 hour after the procedure to prevent soft tissue ischemia post-auricularly and over the hyoid region. Suction drains are removed the morning after surgery unless significant subplatysmal/submandibular gland contouring has been done, in which case drains can remain up to 4 days. In addition, prevention of postoperative nausea and vomiting, as well as pain management, minimize hematoma occurrence.

Recently the senior author (T.G.O'D.) has substituted drain use with the application of a hemostatic net to prevent hematomas in the first 48 hours post-operatively. The net was described in 2014 by Auersvald and Auersvald[13] as a novel technique to essentially eliminate hematoma formation in the early high-risk postoperative period. The indications and experience of the senior author (T.G.O.D.) are well documented in a recently published study.[14] The application of a hemostatic net to all areas of skin elevation to close the dead space by suturing the skin to the deep underlying tissues with a continuous running suture negates the potential of expansive bleeding. The net is accomplished using a Mononylon 5-0 suture with triangular needle of at least 20 mm in length (**Fig. 3**). The hemostatic net is removed on the second post-operative day to prevent marks from the net.

Infection

Owing to the robust vascularity of the face, infection remains a rare occurrence in rhytidectomy and neck lift. When they occur, infections are predominately in the neck. Infection rates have been estimated between at 0.2% and 0.6%.[15]

Infections usually present between postoperative day 5 and 7 and can be rapid and fulminant in presentation. Patients often complain of increased pain and swelling in the submental area (or wherever the infection is located). Local tenderness, fluctuance, erythema, and increased localized swelling are common findings. The infections are usually confined to the preplatysmal plane. Infections need to be treated expeditiously to prevent progression as well as to prevent long-term consequences, including delayed healing, subcutaneous scarring, hospitalization, skin loss, contour irregularities from fat loss, and seroma formation (**Fig. 4**).

In assessing risk factors, in a large cohort of rhytidectomy patients, having a body mass index (BMI) greater than 25 (overweight) and undergoing combined procedures such as concurrent blepharoplasty and brow lift were factors associated with infection.[16] Gender, smoking, diabetes, and age greater than 70 years were not found to be significant risk factors for infection.

A plausible reason why BMI greater than 25 is a risk factor for infection is that these patients require much more lipocontouring and the combination of loose, dead fat cells, blood, and limited neck vascularity explain the increase likelihood of infection. Because *Staphylococcus* and *Streptococcus* are the most common pathogens, allergy or sensitivity to penicillin/cephalosporins also increases risk of infection. Other organisms to be aware of in reticent infections are mouth flora and, rarely, atypical *Mycobacterium* (persistent granuloma).

Intraoperatively, the authors use prophylactic antibiotics and lavage the neck through the submental incision with multiple saline irrigations and betadine solution before neck skin closure. If extensive cautery is used, we irrigate with cool saline solution to reduce heat-related, late microtissue necrosis.

If signs of an infection are ambiguous, warm compresses to increase circulation and close follow-up are the protocol. Once an infection is evident, needle aspiration for Gram stain and culture is done and the infection is needle aspirated. If the abscess is too thick or the infection fulminant, a stab incision is made in a skin crease in order to evacuate the material and irrigate the cavity with diluted betadine. The cavity can then be packed with iodine gauze if necessary.

It is important to remove the infected material because it is acidic and will cause fat necrosis in

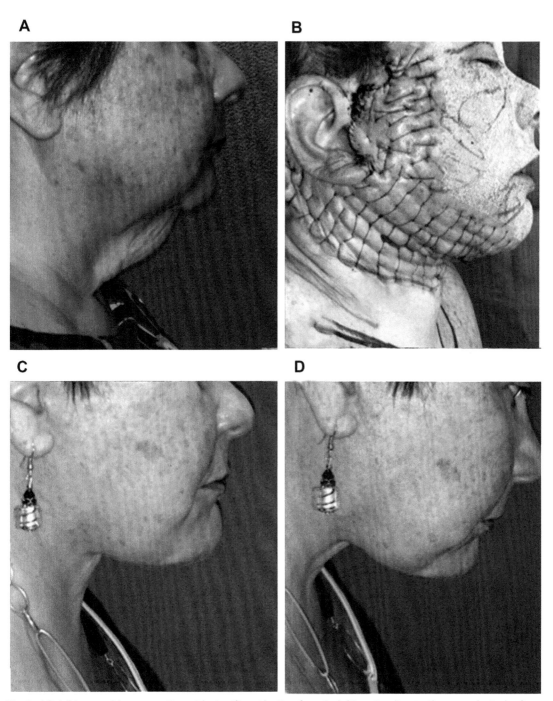

Fig. 3. (*A*) A 64-year-old preoperative with significant laxity of cervical skin extending to the supraclavicular fossa. (*B*) Immediately postoperative after reduction of subplatysmal fat, digastric muscle, and submandibular glands, with redraping of skin to the clavicles. The net prevents hematoma and assists in redistribution of the significantly lax skin. (*C*) Seven months postoperative showing improvement in neck contours and skin redistribution. (*D*) Seven-month Connell views. Procedure performed by T. Gerald O'Daniel, MD, FACS. (*Courtesy of* T. Gerald O'Daniel, MD, FACS, O'Daniel Plastic Surgery Studios, Louisville, KY.)

the region, leading to scarring and an eventual contour defect once the infection resolves.

If the patient is penicillin allergic and the infection significant, the authors treat with intravenous vancomycin for 1 to 5 days, as indicated. If the patient is not penicillin allergic, we treat with Augmentin until cultures dictate the causative organism and their sensitivities to antibiotics.

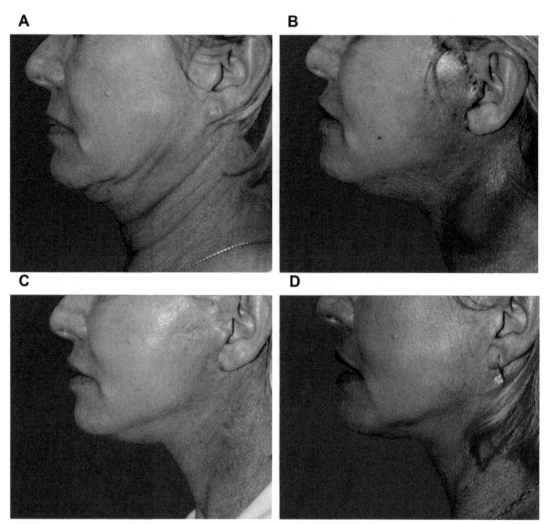

Fig. 4. (*A*) A 59-year-old preoperative for secondary facelift, the primary facelift was done elsewhere. (*B*) One-week postoperative facelift with fat injection and a lateral skin-platysma displacement neck lift presenting with left neck infection. (*C*) Twenty-one days postoperative after drain placement and oral antibiotics. (*D*) Eighteen-month postoperative showing stability of neck lift result and no residual sequela. Secondary procedure performed by T. Gerald O'Daniel, MD, FACS. (*Courtesy of* T. Gerald O'Daniel, MD, FACS, O'Daniel Plastic Surgery Studios, Louisville, KY.)

Seroma

Seroma is a common occurrence in neck lift surgery. The factors that predispose the neck to seroma include wide skin undermining, the dependent nature of the cervical contours, shearing forces between the skin and deep tissues with head movement, and the interruption of lymphatics when subplatysmal surgery is performed. A subcutaneous seroma left untreated can lead to skin ripples, contour irregularities from scarring and weakening of the platysma and superficial cervical fascia, and relapse of muscular laxity. Prevention is key and includes copious irrigation to remove loose fat and serous fluid before closing.

Although the authors only use suction drains overnight, the senior author (T.G.O'D.) utilizes the hemostatic net and restricts head movements in the early post operative period to prevent shearing between the skin and platysma. When subplatysmal surgery is performed, it is advocated that a drain be placed into the subplatysmal space left in place until all drainage stops. T.G.O'D. uses Monocryl as a running deep suture between the platysma and the deep structures to obliterate the dead space lateral to the midline and a running suture to plicate the platysma and the mylohyoid muscle in the midline.

When a seroma occurs, the first treatment is needle aspiration. If there is a recurrence, the

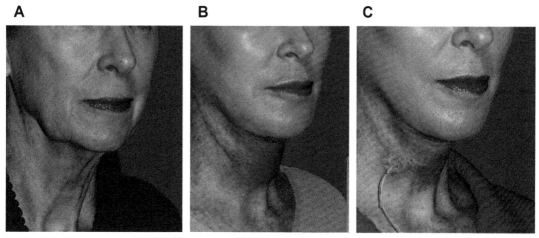

Fig. 5. (*A*) A 68-year-old before facelift and neck lift. (*B*) At 2.5 weeks postoperative seroma, after failed attempts to control with needle aspiration. (*C*) Drain placement that is left in place for 48 hours. Procedure performed by T. Gerald O'Daniel, MD, FACS. (*Courtesy of* T. Gerald O'Daniel, MD, FACS, O'Daniel Plastic Surgery Studios, Louisville, KY.)

authors have a low threshold to treat more aggressively with closed drainage system (**Fig. 5**) or with the application of a hemostatic net.

If a contour irregularity occurs from a seroma, we treat these early with dilute Kenalog injections (4 mg/mL) and aggressive massage by the patient. This treatment resolves most of the issues related to seroma-induced contour irregularities.

Scars

All surgical wounds result in scar formation, but an optimal scar is characterized by being flat, thin, and with excellent color match to the surrounding skin. Incision planning is also an important component of an optimal scar. Incisions should be placed in inconspicuous locations with care to minimize the aesthetic impact on natural focal points such

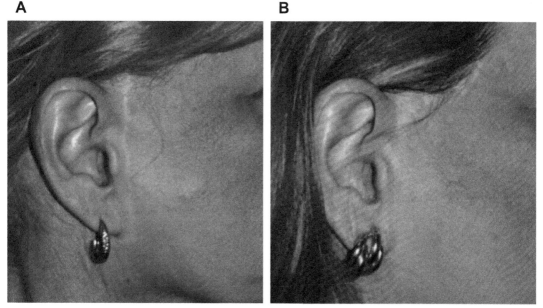

Fig. 6. (*A*) Visible scar secondary to poorly designed facelift incisions from an outside clinic. (*B*) A secondary facelift was performed with the incision design changed to a well-camouflaged retrotragal position with preservation of the infratragal hollow. Secondary procedure performed by T. Gerald O'Daniel, MD, FACS. (*Courtesy of* T. Gerald O'Daniel, MD, FACS, O'Daniel Plastic Surgery Studios, Louisville, KY.)

A **B**

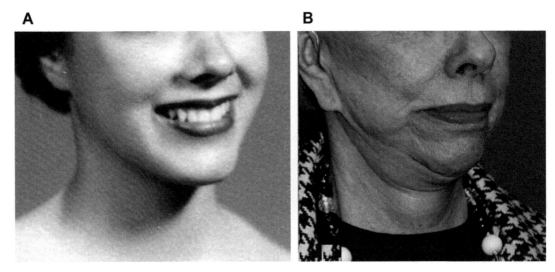

Fig. 7. (*A*) Patient at age 22 years. (*B*) Same patient at age 66 years after a face and supraplatysmal neck lift performed at an outside clinic. Note the excessive tension that created an elongated and distorted earlobe. The line of tension is evident the length of the mandible. The subplatysmal structures have become obvious with the extreme tension. (Pictures used with permission T. Gerald O'Daniel MD, FACS).

as the lobule cheek junction and tragus. Incision designs that fail to respect these principles lead to scar that are conspicuous (**Fig. 6**). When an open neck approach is used, the authors recommend placing the incision posterior to the cervicomental crease to avoid scar depression within the crease, where there is an absence of subcutaneous fat. The incision may be moved as far posteriorly as within 1.5 cm anterior to the hyoid if significant subplatysmal surgery is planned.

Proper surgical technique is a critical component of producing favorable scars. Incisions that are closed under excessive skin tension can lead to unsightly scars, tissue distortions, and lightning of adjacent skin (**Fig. 7**). Skin tension in neck lifting procedures can be minimized by off-loading the tension onto the underlying SMAS fascial layer, and avoiding over-resection of the skin. If a procedure requires skin tension, then a suboptimal scar is likely to be the consequence. In addition to minimizing tension, wound eversion has also been found to result in superior scar cosmesis compared with planar repair, which can result in a more depressed, conspicuous appearance.[17] In addition, avoidance of wound complications such as hematoma, seroma, skin slough, and infection, as discussed elsewhere in this article, is key to a favorable outcome.

Although surgical technique is a major determinant of the mature scar, postoperative wound care continues to exert an effect long after the last suture is in place. Evidence-based methods of preventing hypertrophic scarring include silicone sheeting or silicone gel and hypoallergenic microporous paper tape.[18]

The positive action of silicone is thought to be from inhibition of fibroblasts via its hydration effect.[19] Where avoidance of sun exposure and massage will optimize scar formation, onion extract and vitamin E lotions are commonly used but have unproven clinical efficacy for scar prevention and treatment.[19]

If a suboptimal scar exists, scar revision is an acceptable solution unless the scar is caused by excess skin tension. If scar revision is attempted in this circumstance, then further tension will be created, worsening the outcome. Soft tissue recruitment techniques are necessary to improve scars caused by tension.

Ear Deformity

One of the most blatant signs of a neck lift or facelift is distorted ears and/or conspicuous scars (**Fig. 8**). The success or failure of the procedure is often judged by the aesthetics of the ear scars. In addition to the previously discussed issues of incision planning and tension, an additional issue in the recreation of the original ear shape is understanding how to recreate precise ear anatomy once released by making the initial incision.

When planning the ear incision, both pretragal and retrotragal incisions can be well hidden. In men, because of posterior displacement of the beard line, a pretragal incision is preferred. This

A   **B**

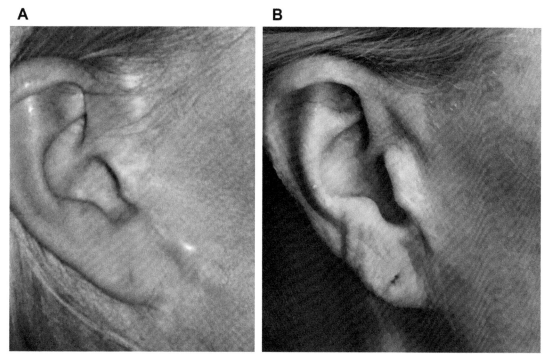

Fig. 8. (*A*) Hypertrophic scars with earlobe and tragal deformities secondary to excessive tension on the skin closure from a facelift performed 2 years previously at an outside clinic. (*B*) Well-healed scars with restoration of the tragus and earlobe 2 years after secondary facelift using a high lamellar SMAS technique to relieve the tension on the skin closure. Procedure performed by T. Gerald O'Daniel, MD, FACS. (*Courtesy of* T. Gerald O'Daniel, MD, FACS, O'Daniel Plastic Surgery Studios, Louisville, KY.)

option should also be considered if the procedure will produce any skin tension in order to avoid anterior displacement of the tragus. If a retrotragal incision is being used, the incision should be placed directly on the edge of the tragus. If the incision is anterior, it will be visible; if it is posterior, it can cause blunting of the sharp edge of the tragus.

Because the earlobe changes position once released by the initial incision, precise recreation of ear anatomy can be more challenging. Having preoperative photographs available to compare the detailed anatomy and positioning of the earlobe is essential. In addition, careful observation of the earlobe while the patient is in the surgical position reveals details of positioning that may differ from the photographs and will not be evident once the incision is made.

Tension on the skin closure not only distorts the tragus but the earlobe is also affected. The most obvious sign of a facelift or neck lift is an elongated or distorted earlobe. When obvious, it is called a pixie ear deformity, and this is often associated with hypertrophic scars and keloids, particularly in genetically predisposed patients (**Fig. 9**).

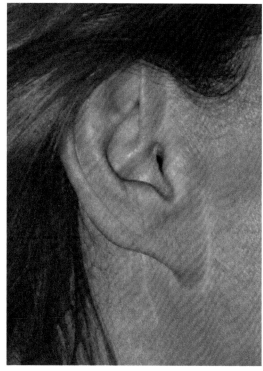

Fig. 9. An elongated lobule creating a pixie ear deformity. (*Courtesy of* N. Gordon, MD, FACS, Wilton, CT.)

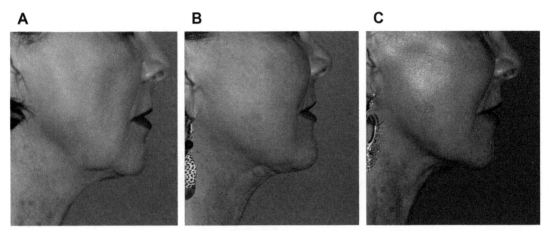

Fig. 10. (A) A 59-year-old patient seen preoperatively for secondary face and neck lift. (B) Postoperatively she has redundant skin in the submental region. (C) An elliptical excision of the redundant skin creates a smooth and pleasing surface. Procedure performed by T. Gerald O'Daniel, MD, FACS. (*Courtesy of* T. Gerald O'Daniel, MD, FACS, O'Daniel Plastic Surgery Studios, Louisville, KY.)

If mild earlobe elongation exists, this can be improved with a V-Y advancement, which repositions the earlobe superiorly but leaves a longer scar inferior to the lobe. If a significant pixie ear deformity exists and is associated with hypertrophic scars, the soft tissue defect and resultant tension require recruitment of additional soft tissue. This recruitment can be accomplished by revision rhytidectomy, in which tension can be released and additional soft tissue used to recreate the native anatomy without tension. Simple scar revision makes the soft tissue deficit worse and can lead to an exacerbation of both the pixie ear and hypertrophic scarring and should be avoided.

Skin Loss

Because surgery for neck rejuvenation involves separation of the skin from the platysma muscle and creates a long random flap, complication related to skin injury is common and has an incidence of 3% to 5%.[20] The area that is most vulnerable is the postauricular region, especially if closed under tension.

Patients with medical conditions, such as diabetes mellitus, and nicotine users are predisposed to ischemic issues even if there are no other surgical issues such as tension. Other causes can be overly aggressive liposuction causing injury to the subdermal vascular plexus, cautery of the skin flap, or an excessively tight dressing. An ischemic area of the skin flap can start innocuously as a small area of epidermal sloughing and then can progress to full-thickness tissue loss. Because the flap is random and poorly vascularized, healing of even a small full-thickness injury can progress

very slowly and leave a poor circumferential scar. Avoidance of flap cautery and overaggressive liposuction is clearly preferable, and, if an area of the flap appears potentially ischemic during or after surgery, small applications of nitroglycerin ointment 2% can prevent further ischemic injury. Postoperatively, if a larger area of tissue appears to be ischemic, hyperbaric oxygen treatments can be effective in reversing the ischemic process and maximizing tissue salvage.

If an area of skin shows full-thickness tissue loss, excision of an ellipse and closure of healthy tissue can be most effective. Although acceptable, the authors do not find aggressive marginal tissue debridement advisable. This technique often leads to a larger area of depigmented scar than maximizing oxygenation and keeping the wound moist with topicals such as Vaseline or Silvadene and healing by secondary intention.

Redundant Skin

Issues of redundant skin occur most commonly in procedures that tighten underlying soft tissue without removing skin excess. Redundant skin can also occur when the soft tissue tightening is greater than the skin tightening. This problem can also occur as a later aesthetic issue when a closed neck procedure was accomplished and the patient ages and exposes the corrected deep, soft tissue without the corresponding skin adjustment.

If the skin redundancy is limited, treatment can include direct excision in a skin crease using an elliptical design (**Fig. 10**). If significant and a result of neck lift, then the flaps may need to be raised

A

B

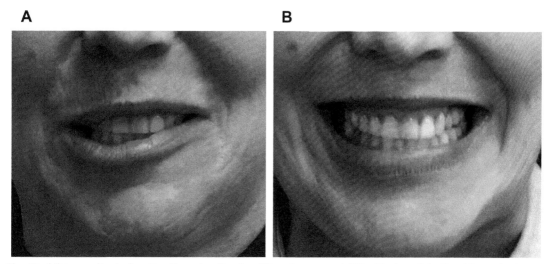

Fig. 11. (*A*) Lower lip dysfunction 2 weeks after facelift and open neck lift with deep fat, digastric, and submandibular gland reduction. Note the elevated left lip from paramedian depressor dysfunction from either the depressor inferioris or platysma pars labialis paresis. The depressor anguli oris is fully functional. (*B*) Three months postoperative with complete return of function. Procedure performed by T. Gerald O'Daniel, MD, FACS. (*Courtesy of* T. Gerald O'Daniel, MD, FACS, O'Daniel Plastic Surgery Studios, Louisville, KY.)

and redraped or a facelift/neck lift accomplished in cases in which only a past limited procedure was done.

Nerve Injury

The most common motor disturbance of facial musculature in neck lift surgery is related to an asymmetrical smile from disruption of depressor function of the lower lip. The cause of this deformity may be an injury to the cervical or marginal mandibular branches of the facial nerve or an injury to the platysma.[21,22] The lower lip deformity is typically characterized by a lack of downward motion of the paramedian lower lip and often an upward rise of the lip margin on the affected side as well. This deformity corresponds with dysfunction of the depressor labii inferioris or the platysma pars labialis. In one author's (T.G.O'D.) experience, there was 1.5% lower lip dysfunction out of 247 facelifts and neck lifts over the last 24 months. All patients recovered between 1 week and 3 months (**Fig. 11**). Watchful waiting is prudent in cases of lower lip dysfunction because complete recovery is expected. If a patient finds the lip dysfunction overly bothersome, a neuromodulator can be injected into the contralateral unaffected paramedian depressor muscles to create a symmetric smile until the injury resolves (**Fig. 12**). The injection of a neuromodulator into the contralateral unaffected lip leads to bilateral elevation of the lower lip on smiling, creating a Mona Lisa smile in which the lower teeth are not revealed.

A

B

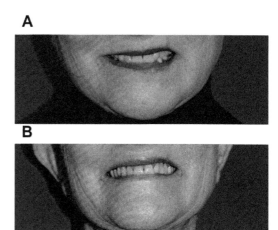

Fig. 12. (*A*) Lower lip dysfunction 2 weeks after facelift and open neck lift with deep fat, digastric, and submandibular gland reduction. Note the elevated right lip from paramedian depressor dysfunction from either the depressor inferioris or platysma pars labialis paresis. The depressor anguli oris is fully functional. (*B*) After botulinum neuromodulator injectors into the left unaffected paramedian depressor musculature. Note the bilateral symmetric lower lip elevation creating a Mona Lisa smile that does not show the lower teeth. A single injection was needed until complete recovery occurred. Procedure performed by T. Gerald O'Daniel, MD, FACS. (*Courtesy of* T. Gerald O'Daniel, MD, FACS, O'Daniel Plastic Surgery Studios, Louisville, KY.)

Supraplatysma Fat Deformities

The fat in the supraplatysma plane is the most often addressed component of the aging neck. This fat is commonly reduced with suction-assisted lipectomy or direct lipectomy. Deformities can be created from irregular resection, over-resection, and under-resection.

Over-resection of supraplatysma fat can occur with any approach to the neck. Fat resection is done as a maneuver to create an optimal neck contour but in the aging neck multiple factors often contribute to an obtuse, heavy-appearing neck, with supraplatysma fat being only 1 of the components. In addition, because the supraplatysma space is easily accessed, the combination of misdiagnosis and ease of access leads to over-resection, which can lead to contour irregularities, skeletonization of the platysma revealing platysma bands, platysma movement, and visible subplatysmal structures that were previously hidden by the subcutaneous fat.

Contour irregularities can occur when the transition from the thicker jawline fat to neck fat is too severe. This condition often occurs when the reduction of neck volume is overzealous in the supraplatysmal plane in the effort to create an acute cervicomental angle. The only correction of this deformity is to add volume back to the subcutaneous plane with microfat grafting, which is an inconsistent solution.

In addition, when the subcutaneous fat is deficient, the platysma adherent to the skin can be seen. At rest there may not be an obvious deformity; however, on animation the platysmal contraction is overly visible (**Fig. 13**). Correction of this deformity is difficult, with the only solution being microfat grafting to add volume back to the subcutaneous plane.

Contour irregularities can result from an uneven resection of the supraplatysma fat (**Fig. 14**). When raising the neck flaps, clinicians should leave approximately 5 mm of subcutaneous fat attached to the undersurface of the skin. The fat that remains on the platysma should be removed evenly from the platysma, taking care to leave the superficial cervical fascia intact. Injury to the superficial cervical fascia overlying the platysma can also lead to contour irregularities caused by the bulges of the muscle in areas of fascial damage, as well as revealing subplatysmal structures. Intraoperatively during an open neck procedure, running a finger on the flap to ensure even fat distribution is helpful to avoid irregularities, which could require secondary operations to create the desired smooth cervical contour.

Platysma

Recurrent platysma bands

Nothing typifies the aged neck and motivates people to seek solutions better than ptotic, platysma bands. A unique muscle, the platysma is invested with the superficial cervical fascia of the head and neck, extending from the fascia of the pectoralis major inferiorly to the body of the mandible and extending cephalad by incorporating into the SMAS of the midface. As the

A   B

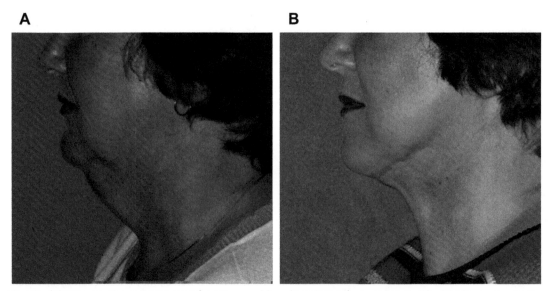

Fig. 13. (*A*) Preoperative appearance of a 55-year-old undergoing a face and neck lift. (*B*) The postoperative appearance from over-resection of supraplatysmal fat showing the concavity along the jawline.

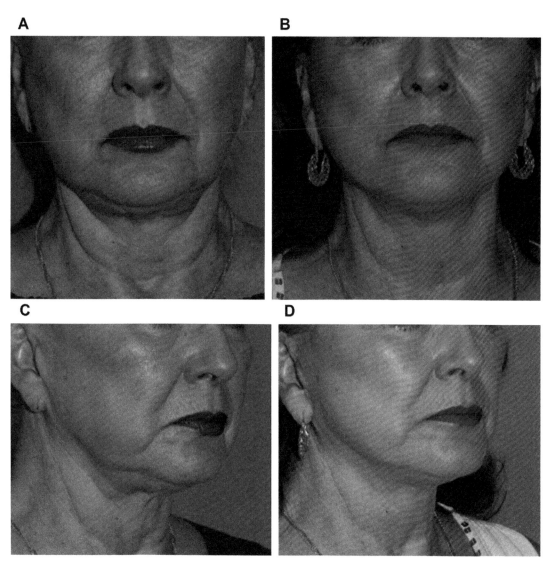

Fig. 14. (A) Front and (C) side views of preoperative appearance of a 69-year-old undergoing a secondary neck lift for irregular supraplatysma fat. (B) Front and (D) side views of the postoperative appearance at 70 years of age, 1 year postoperatively after revision of neck lift to create a smooth submental surface and improved jawline. Procedure performed by T. Gerald O'Daniel, MD, FACS. (*Courtesy of* T. Gerald O'Daniel, MD, FACS, O'Daniel Plastic Surgery Studios, Louisville, KY.)

underbelly of the superficial soft tissue envelope of the midface and neck, it is the boundary between superficial soft tissue and deeper, structural aspects of the face and neck. Because it is part of the superficial soft tissue envelope and not attached to fixed points as most muscles are, the platysma is a marker of the gravitational aging effects in the midface and neck. The restoration of a youthful neckline depends on adequate treatment of platysma banding more than any other neck feature, and failure of treatment is a common complaint in seeking further modalities or revision surgery.

Effective treatment of platysmal bands requires appropriate diagnosis and differentiation of the type of band present.[23] Platysmal bands can be either adynamic redundant muscles associated with loose skin or they may be dynamic bands that become more apparent on animation. Asking these patients to tighten their neck muscles while pushing the jaw forward and showing their lower teeth with a grimace activates the platysma. Treatments differ for either type of band. If the bands are adynamic and redundant, an anterior platysmaplasty can reduce the horizontal laxity and restore the cervicomental angle. When dynamic bands are present, the platysmaplasty alone cannot be expected to effectively treat platysma bands. The dynamic bands are most often medially located but there can also be lateral dynamic bands. Successful treatment can be accomplished with platysma myotomy. If the patient has isolated anterior medial dynamic bands, the myotomy is placed low in the anterior neck at the level of the cricoid cartilage. If there is also an associated lateral band, then a complete platysma myotomy is performed by connecting the medial transection with the lateral myotomy placed low in the lateral neck.

Platysma treatment failures often present as recurrent or persistent platysma bands. Either type of band can recur. Recurrence can be an immediate aesthetic issue or occur many months after surgery[24] (**Fig. 15**). The causes are diverse. Causes can be as simple as undertreatment of the platysma muscle leaving ptotic muscle still evident. Because the platysma is often suture embrocated, another cause is failure of embrocation either because of sutures pulling through the muscle or related to other causes, such as hematoma or seroma, which can weaken the muscle fixation and lead to dehiscence. In addition, failure can be related to the failure to properly differentiate the type of platysma band preoperatively, with subsequent failure to properly perform a myotomy for dynamic platysma bands.

In these situations, direct treatment of the recurrent or persistent platysma can cure the issue. Further resection and/or resuture embrocation is necessary (**Figs. 16** and **17**). If recurrence is caused by sutures failing, then a more significant fixation, such as a corset embrocation, may be more effective. When the recurrence is caused by undertreatment of a dynamic platysma band, temporary relief can be achieved with injection of a neuromodulator. Definitive treatment can be accomplished with a partial or complete myotomy that effectively divides the band (**Figs. 18** and **19**).

Another cause of posttreatment platysma banding is misdiagnosis, such as a ptotic platysma being present preprocedure and it not being addressed. This situation often occurs in the post–50-year-old heavy neck in which lipectomy/liposuction is the sole treatment modality. The platysma bands were hidden in the heavy neck and exposed when the fat was removed. The authors are now also seeing a similar concept with minimally invasive energy devices, in which the devices mainly tighten skin and destroy the

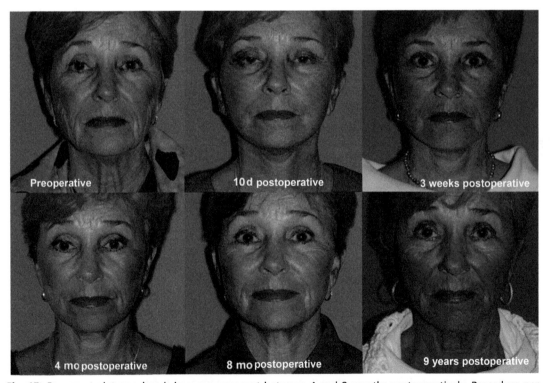

Fig. 15. Recurrent platysma bands become apparent between 4 and 8 months postoperatively. Procedure performed by T. Gerald O'Daniel, MD, FACS. (*Courtesy of* T. Gerald O'Daniel, MD, FACS, O'Daniel Plastic Surgery Studios, Louisville, KY.)

A

B

C

D

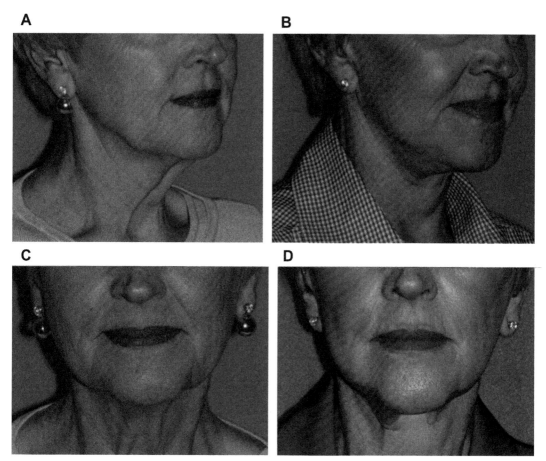

Fig. 16. (*A*) Side and (*C*) front views of a 62-year-old preoperative facelift and platysma plication. (*B*) One year postoperatively with presumed platysma plication failure. (*D*) At 4 years postoperatively, with obvious bands. Procedure performed by T. Gerald O'Daniel, MD, FACS. (*Courtesy of* T. Gerald O'Daniel, MD, FACS, O'Daniel Plastic Surgery Studios, Louisville, KY.)

supraplatysmal fat, and this often exposes otherwise hidden platysma bands and requires direct treatment to eliminate.

Inadequate treatment of digastric muscles can be confused with persistent platysma banding. In this case, the fixated platysma can be palpated midline and the ptotic neck structure is paramedian and travels inferolateral to the lateral aspect of the hyoid bone. Careful preoperative assessment can prevent this occurrence and direct treatment of the digastric muscle solves this issue.

In addition, a common and often overlooked cause is failure in midface lifting. Because the platysma muscle is the underbelly of the superficial soft tissue envelope and gravity's effects chiefly influence this anatomic unit, this leads to stretching and elongating until the characteristic redundant, aged neck is created. If the midface is inadequately repositioned, persistent or recurrent platysma bands will be evident. Aggressive platysma

resection and embrocation do not cure this issue and often revision rhytidectomy is necessary to reposition the platysma superolaterally.[9]

Deformity from Platysma Myotomy

Attempts to prevent recurrent platysma bands can themselves create deformities. When there are active platysmal bands it is advocated in some circumstances to perform a complete platysma myotomy. The platysma myotomy is a very effective method to disrupt dynamic platysma bands as well as to allow release of the platysma in short necks. Although any platysma myotomy can theoretically become apparent, when a platysma myotomy is placed too superior, a secondary deformity characterized by herniation of the submandibular triangle contents can occur. Management of this deformity requires repair of the myotomy and potential management of the submandibular triangle

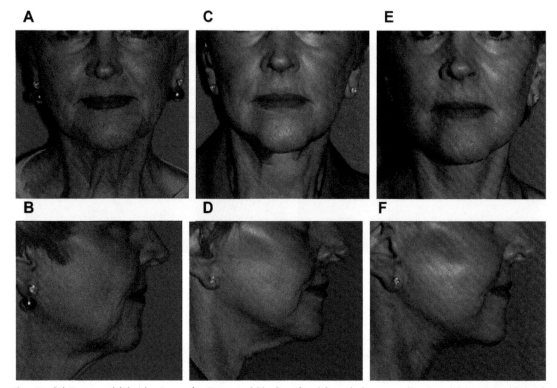

Fig. 17. (*A*) Front and (*B*) side views of a 62-year-old before facelift and platysma plication. (*C*) Front and (*D*) side views 4 years postoperatively of recurrent bands after platysma plication failure. (*E*) Front and (*F*) side views 6 years after secondary repair, which included mobilization of the platysma and a platysma corset performed with a low myotomy at the level of the cricoid cartilage. At the secondary surgery, the initial plication was intact and the recurrent bands were newly formed at the edge of the central myotomy. Procedure performed by T. Gerald O'Daniel, MD, FACS. (*Courtesy of* T. Gerald O'Daniel, MD, FACS, O'Daniel Plastic Surgery Studios, Louisville, KY.)

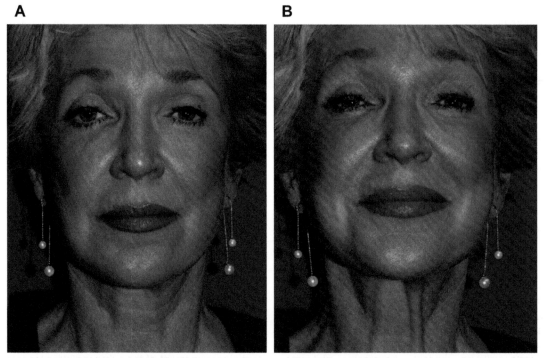

Fig. 18. (*A*) A 59-year-old 1 year after primary facelift elsewhere presenting with recurrent bands. (*B*) On animation the dynamic bands are obvious.

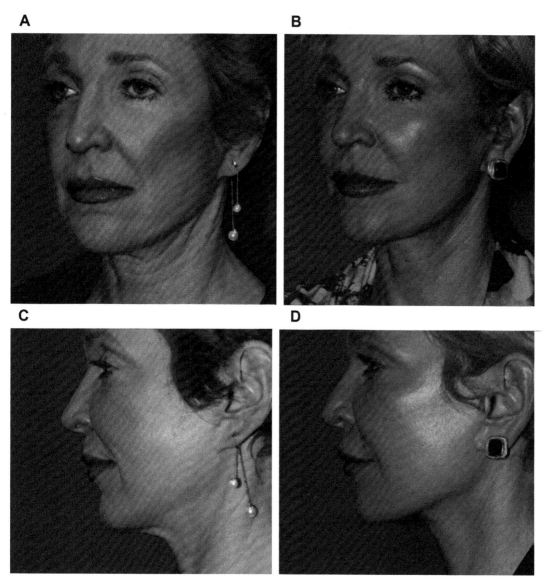

Fig. 19. (*A*) Front and (*C*) side views of a 59-year-old 1 year after facelift performed elsewhere presenting with recurrent bands. (*B*) Front and (*D*) side views of 1 year after secondary facelift with anterior platysmaplasty and complete platysma myotomy. Microfat injection and a reverse brow lift were also performed. Procedure performed by T. Gerald O'Daniel, MD, FACS. (*Courtesy of* T. Gerald O'Daniel, MD, FACS, O'Daniel Plastic Surgery Studios, Louisville, KY.)

contents, including medial and lateral extensions of the subplatysmal fat and submandibular glands (**Fig. 20**).

Central Neck Deformities Related to the Subplatysmal Structures

Surgery that addresses the subplatysmal structures (subplatysmal fat, digastric muscle, perihyoid fascia, and the submandibular glands) is not commonly performed. The surgery required to address these structures demands that the surgeon work through a small submental incision on structures that are distant from the incision and in a confined space. Subplatysmal surgery takes additional time, and the increased complexity of the procedure exposes the patient to increased risk, including contour irregularities, seromas, sialoceles, injury to the cervical branch of the facial nerve, and arterial bleeding.[25] However, the risk of not addressing these structures is a less-than-optimal outcome related to persistent central/

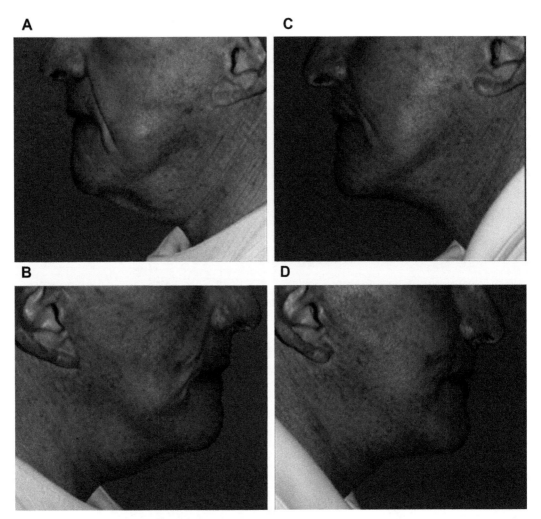

Fig. 20. (*A*) Left side and (*B*) right-side views 10 years after platysma myotomy results in herniation of subman-dibular contents. The primary facelift and neck lift was performed elsewhere. (*C*) Left side and (*D*) right-side views of 1-year postoperative repair of platysma myotomy, management of submandibular triangle contents, platysma-plasty, and secondary facelift. Secondary procedure performed by T. Gerald O'Daniel, MD, FACS. (*Courtesy of* T. Gerald O'Daniel, MD, FACS, O'Daniel Plastic Surgery Studios, Louisville, KY.)

paramedian neck deformities or deformities made worse by the overzealous attempts to create a pleasing cervicomental angle by addressing only the platysma and supraplatysmal fat (**Fig. 21**).

It is helpful to think of the deep neck anatomy as the submental triangle and the submandibular tri-angle. The submental triangle is the central aspect of the neck; its borders are the anterior digastric muscles and its base is the hyoid bone. The roof of the submental triangle is the mylohyoid muscle. The central fat pad of the subplatysmal fat is con-tained within the submental triangle. The perihyoid fascia also is at the base of the triangle and in some instances is thickened and significantly con-tributes to the cervicomental angle. The submandibular triangle is in a paramedian position and its borders are the anterior and posterior digastric muscle and the mandibular border. Con-tained within this triangle are the medial and lateral extensions of the deep subplatysmal fat and the submandibular gland.

Because many surgeons do not approach sub-platysmal structures in neck surgery, it is imperative to accurately diagnose these issues preoperatively and make the patient aware that this region of the neck will not be treated. In addition, the surgeon must factor the lack of central/paramedian neck treatment in the treatment of the more commonly treated median regions to avoid imbalances and suboptimal aesthetic results.

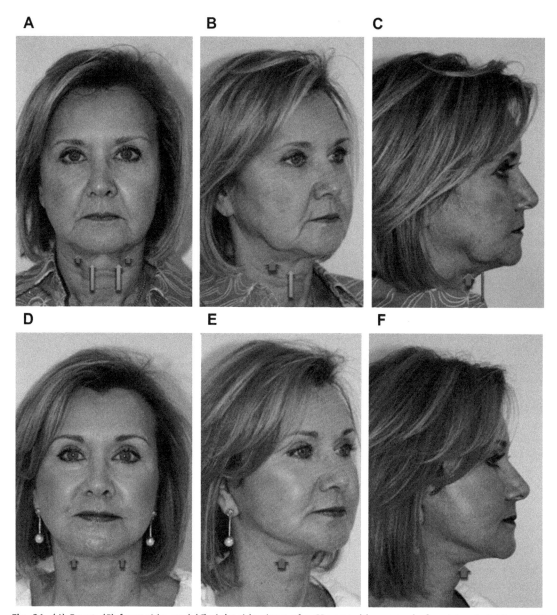

Fig. 21. (A) Front, (B) front-side, and (C) right-side views of a 62-year-old woman before tricophytal brow lift, deep-plane rhytidectomy, with buccal fat resection. The blue arrows define the ptotic platysma muscle, red arrows define the ptotic submandibular gland and digastric muscle. (D) Front, (E) front-side, and (F) right-side postoperative views. Note the persistence of paramedian neck fullness caused by failure of submandibular gland and digastric muscle. The patient was satisfied and did not seek further treatment. Procedure performed by Neil A. Gordon, MD. (*Courtesty of* Neil A. Gordon, MD, Wilton, Conn.)

Submental Triangle Deformities

An obtuse cervicomental angle can be present at a young age and is often a presenting complaint when young patients wish to improve their profiles. In aging patients seeking facial rejuvenation, the goal of treatment is typically to restore the past facial appearance. Often an aging facial profile is complicated by a preexisting obtuse cervicomental angle that has worsened with the aging process because of a greater accumulation of subplatysmal fat, digastric muscle enlargement, and submandibular gland enlargement that cannot be contained in the aging mandibular skeletal confines.

In cases in which the goal is to improve native neck contours, whether during aging face treatment or in younger patients seeking isolated

A   B   C

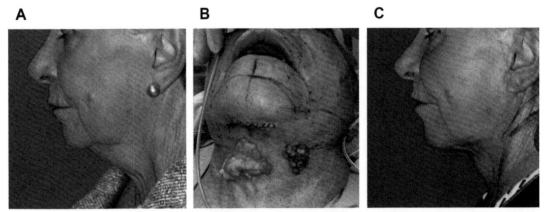

Fig. 22. (*A*) A 69-year-old patient 10 years after extended SMAS facelift and supraplatysmal fat reduction with suction-assisted lipectomy. (*B*) Intraoperative view during a secondary open neck lift with reduction of the sub-platysmal fat and left submandibular gland. (*C*) One year after isolated neck lift with management of the sub-platysmal fat and submandibular glands. Procedure performed by T. Gerald O'Daniel, MD, FACS. (*Courtesy of* T. Gerald O'Daniel, MD, FACS, O'Daniel Plastic Surgery Studios, Louisville, KY.)

neck improvement, the cervicomental angle can remain an issue after the procedure, limit the extent of neck improvement, and cause dissatisfaction if this was an intended goal and the offending anatomic structures are not addressed.

The subplatysmal fat is the major factor in central neck fullness. To understand the impact of this fat, a typical example of the impact of ignoring the deep fat on the initial operation is shown in **Fig. 22**. The first operation was a lateral-only approach with aggressive supraplatysmal fat removal with suction-assisted lipectomy and extensive lateral release of facial ligaments and platysma with a deep SMAS facelift. Secondary operation revealed the cause of the obtuse angle, which was the failure to address the subplatysmal fat and submandibular glands.

The management of one structure without attention to the adjacent structures can create new contour irregularities and even create significant deformities. For instance, because of ease of access, aggressive reduction of subplatysmal fat without management of the more challenging paramedian structures (digastric muscles and submandibular glands) may create an exaggerated central neck convexity if the subplatysmal fat is not treated in a conservative fashion. This deformity is referred to as a cobra deformity and is obvious at rest and made more noticeable on flexion of the platysmal muscle. Correction requires the subplatysmal space to be reentered and the paramedian fullness addressed by management of the digastric muscles with reduction and possible digastric plication to restore volume in the deep central neck, possible reduction of the medial and lateral extensions of the

subplatysmal fat, and also possible reduction of the submandibular gland (**Fig. 23**). Prevention of a cobra deformity is 2-fold. First, if the surgeon is not committed to addressing the paramedian fullness, then it is imperative that the subplatysmal fat only be reduced to the plane even with the central bulge of the digastric muscle. The second method of prevention is to address the paramedian structures.

The second structure that may contribute to an obtuse cervicomental angle is at the base of the submental triangle, and this is the perihyoid fascia. Failure to release or possibly resect the fascia in cases of anteriorly positioned hyoid can lead to a failure to achieve an ideal cervicomental angle. In some instances, the perihyoid fascia may be the sole contributor to a failed neck lift. **Fig. 24** shows a 69-year-old patient who had a previous subplatysmal surgery during a secondary face and neck lift. The persistence of a blunted cervicomental angle was the result of a failure to adequately address the perihyoid fascia in the secondary operation. Resection of the fascia and a plication of the platysma into the new contours achieved a pleasing cervicomental angle.

Paramedian Fullness: Anterior Digastric Muscle

The anterior digastric muscle is the transition point from the submental triangle to the submandibular triangle. When a satisfying neck contour is not achieved and the fullness is paramedian, the cause is most likely related to the anterior belly of the digastric muscle. Often confused with platysma banding, correctly diagnosing digastric

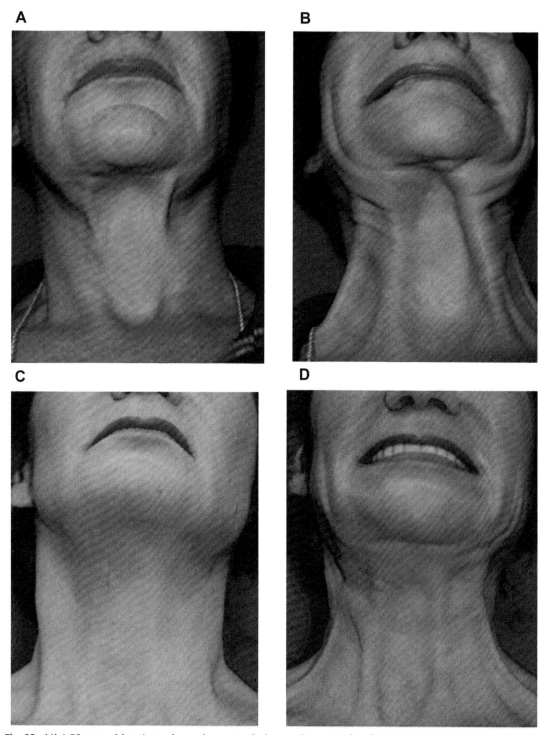

Fig. 23. (*A*) A 58-year-old patient who underwent subplatysmal surgery elsewhere presents with a cobra deformity from over-resection of the subplatysmal fat while ignoring the digastric muscles and submandibular glands. (*B*) The deformity worsens with contraction of the platysma muscle. (*C*) Patient at rest after secondary surgery to correct the deformity, which required reduction of the paramedian volume with partial resection of the anterior digastric muscle and submandibular glands and a platysma plication into the newly created contours. (*D*) Contraction of the platysma shows elimination of the cobra deformity. Secondary procedure performed by T. Gerald O'Daniel, MD, FACS. (*Courtesy of* T. Gerald O'Daniel, MD, FACS, O'Daniel Plastic Surgery Studios, Louisville, KY.)

A   **B**

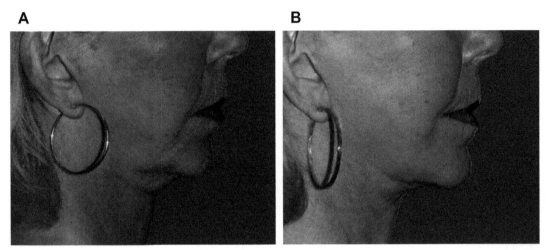

Fig. 24. (*A*) A 68-year-old who is 8 years after secondary facelift and neck lift with subplatysmal surgery. (*B*) One year after tertiary neck lift with perihyoid fascia release/resection with creation of a more ideal cervicomental angle. Secondary procedure performed by T. Gerald O'Daniel, MD, FACS. (*Courtesy of* T. Gerald O'Daniel, MD, FACS, O'Daniel Plastic Surgery Studios, Louisville, KY.)

banding is critical in producing predictable and complete neck lift outcomes. Unlike platysma banding, digastric bands are further paramedian and descend in a tangent inferolateral to the lateral aspect of the hyoid (**Fig. 25**). Although platysma bands can descend inferior to the hyoid, the digastric cannot. The anterior digastric bulge is caused by the central, thickened muscle. Because the submandibular gland sits in the submandibular triangle, gland enlargement is more of a concentric bulge at the hyoid digastric junction (**Fig. 26**).

When the anterior digastric muscle is thickened with a midbelly fullness, then reduction of the central anterior belly resection is necessary to prevent paramedian fullness. The reduction can be done as well in conjunction with the digastric plication. Placing a clamp through the middle of this part of the muscle belly and resecting the central inferior/dependent hanging portion with a unipolar cautery corrects the ptotic digastric muscle.

Submandibular Triangle

The submandibular gland is the main occupant of the submandibular triangle and with the lateral subplatysmal fat pad contributes to the volume within the triangle. Management of the submandibular gland is not widely performed because of the distant position of the gland from the submental incision and because of the significant vascular structures in and around the gland. A careful and precisely planned approach with a complete understanding of the complex anatomy is imperative when reduction of the submandibular gland is

to be performed.[26,27] Often the only way to achieve a well-balanced face and neck is to address the enlarged submandibular gland by reducing the portion of the superficial lobe of the gland that projects past the line drawn from the mandibular border and posterior digastric muscle (**Fig. 27**). The senior author (T.G.O'D.), addresses the submandibular gland in approximately 70% of his neck lifts.

Complications related to submandibular gland resection include inadequate resection, recurrent ptosis, sialocele, bleeding, and injury to the cervical branch of the facial nerve. Inadequate resection can occur when there is insufficient mobilization of the gland and the ability to fully assess the gland is compromised. Widely opening the capsule surrounding the gland and releasing the gland from the surrounding soft tissue generously achieves full mobility of the gland. This mobility significantly improves visualization of the gland, which assists in determining how much gland to resect as well as increasing the surgeon's ability to control any bleeding that may occur during resection. Because a branch of the cervical branch of the facial nerve is outside the lateral capsule, opening the medial capsule and working within the capsule protects the nerve. Injury to a cervical branch of the facial nerve can occur when using unipolar cautery on the anterior capsule because the nerve may lie outside the capsule on the undersurface of the platysma. Care should be taken with cautery in the area to prevent injury. Injuries to the motor nerve are covered earlier.

After resection of the gland, a hemostatic net is placed along the portion of the inferior remnant of

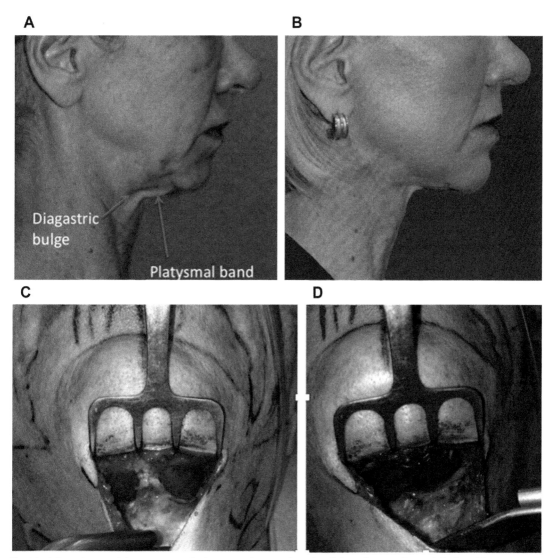

Fig. 25. (*A*) A 58-year-old preoperatively showing platysma band and the adjacent digastric bulge. (*B*) At 9 months after facelift and neck lift, fat injection, and CO_2 laser. The digastric plication elevated the muscle, creating an optimal cervical angle and contour. (*C*) Intraoperative finding shows the digastric bulge before plication. (*D*) After the digastric plication. Note the elevation of the submental triangle and elimination of the digastric bulge. Procedure performed by T. Gerald O'Daniel, MD, FACS. (*Courtesy of* T. Gerald O'Daniel, MD, FACS, O'Daniel Plastic Surgery Studios, Louisville, KY.)

the gland. This 4-0 Monocryl suture, on a large atraumatic needle, is applied as a running suture that compresses the resected surface of the gland to prevent spontaneous bleeding from the central perforating artery. It reduces the raw surface area and assists in controlling the residual shape of the gland. The capsule is then closed with the same suture, by suturing the anterior capsule to the posterior digastric muscle, creating a tight and complete closure of the dead space created from the partial removal of the gland.

Sialocele

Bothersome sialoceles can occur after partial removal of the gland. Preventive measures include injection of a neuromodulator after resection, application of the net, coverage with fibrin glue, and watertight closure of the capsule. Postoperatively the patients are place on a strict low salivary production diet. Before taking these steps, the senior author (T.G.O'D.) experienced sialoceles that were treated with drain placement (**Fig. 28**), injection of a neuromodulator, and use of a scopolamine patch.

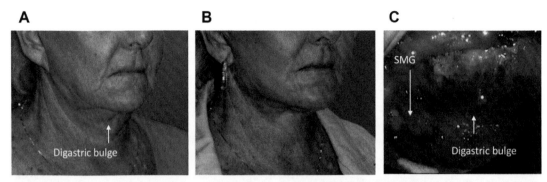

Fig. 26. (A) A 67-year-old who underwent 2 previous open neck supraplatysmal surgeries elsewhere with persistent contour irregularities secondary to the digastric muscle and enlarged submandibular gland. (B) Two years after tertiary face and neck lift with reduction of the digastric muscle and submandibular gland. (C) Intraoperative view of the digastric bulge and enlarged submandibular gland (SMG). Tertiary procedure performed by T. Gerald O'Daniel, MD, FACS. (*Courtesy of* T. Gerald O'Daniel, MD, FACS, O'Daniel Plastic Surgery Studios, Louisville, KY.)

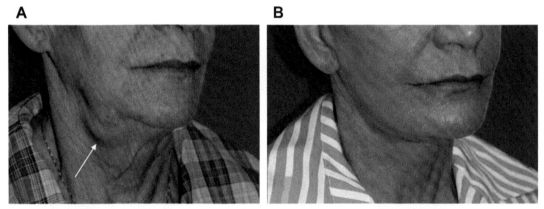

Fig. 27. (A) Preoperative 64-year-old with thin neck and a prominent, enlarged submandibular gland (*arrow*) extending out of the submandibular triangle. (B) One year after face and neck lift with reduction of the superficial lobe of the submandibular gland. Procedure performed by T. Gerald O'Daniel, MD, FACS. (*Courtesy of* T. Gerald O'Daniel, MD, FACS, O'Daniel Plastic Surgery Studios, Louisville, KY.)

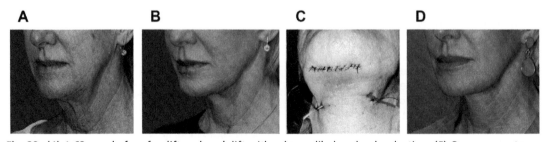

Fig. 28. (A) A 63-year before facelift and neck lift with submandibular gland reduction. (B) One year postoperatively with residual fullness in the submandibular triangle requiring secondary neck lift and further reduction of the gland. (C) Bilateral sialoceles occurred requiring bilateral drain placement. Patient also placed on dietary restrictions, had neuromodulator injections, and wore a scopolamine patch until resolution was achieved. (D) One year after secondary neck lift showing adequate reduction of the residual prominent gland. Procedure performed by T. Gerald O'Daniel, MD, FACS. (*Courtesy of* T. Gerald O'Daniel, MD, FACS, O'Daniel Plastic Surgery Studios, Louisville, KY.)

Nonsurgical Neck Lift Complications

Nonsurgical aesthetic medicine is the fastest-growing segment of people seeking aesthetic procedures, with a 28% to 40% growth from 2012 to 2017.[28] Nonsurgical treatment of the neck and lower face has seen significant growth as patients seek ways to improve the appearance of their necks without the perceived risk, expense, and recovery of a surgical procedure. Industry's rapid technological development and direct-to-consumer marketing has resulted in a large

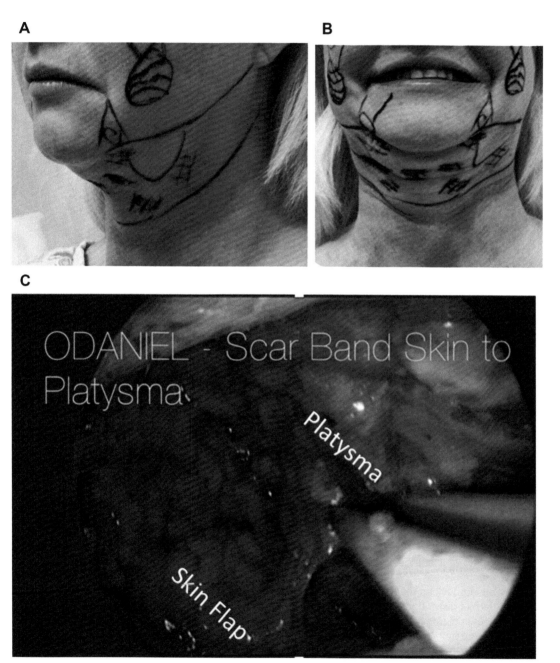

Fig. 29. (*A*) Submental irregularities noted with areas of adhesion that occurred after radiofrequency energy delivery to improve cervical contours and skin laxity. Performed at outside medispa. (*B*) The deformity is accentuated on platysmal contraction. (*C*) Intraoperative view showing one of the adhesion bands extending from the subcutaneous skin to the platysma. Secondary procedure performed by T. Gerald O'Daniel, MD, FACS. (*Courtesy of* T. Gerald O'Daniel, MD, FACS, O'Daniel Plastic Surgery Studios, Louisville, KY.)

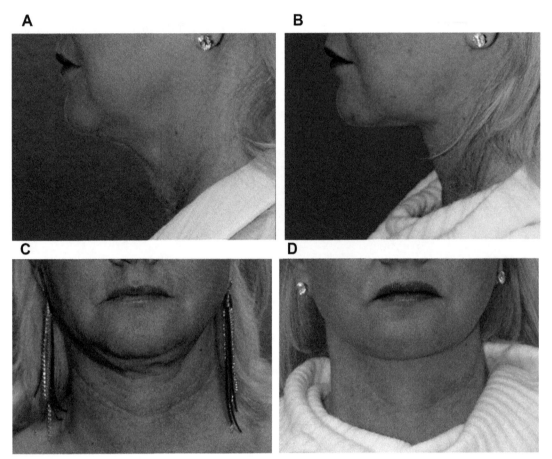

Fig. 30. (*A*) Side and (*C*) front views of preoperative submental irregularities noted with areas of adhesion that occurred after radiofrequency energy delivery to improve cervical contours and skin laxity. Performed at outside medispa. (*B*) Side and (*D*) front views 1 year after facelift with fat injection and open neck procedure to reduce subplatysmal fat, digastric, and submandibular glands. Secondary procedure performed by T. Gerald O'Daniel, MD, FACS. (*Courtesy of* T. Gerald O'Daniel, MD, FACS, O'Daniel Plastic Surgery Studios, Louisville, KY.)

number of patients undergoing a wide variety of treatment, ranging from energy delivery devices to lipocryotherapy and injection of enzymatic agents to reduce the supraplatysmal fat. The efficacies of these treatments are unpredictable at best.

The authors are now starting to treat an assortment of deformities that are created from the indiscriminate nature of tissue destruction that occurs from these technologies.

Energy-based devices that deliver enough heat to cause thermal disruption of collagen fibers can create overheating, uneven loss of the subcutaneous fat, and creation of scars between the skin and muscle. These patients present a new subset of complications that may have particularly difficult solutions. **Figs. 29** and **30** show the typical deformity encountered after delivery of transcutaneous thermal energy that creates uneven loss of supraplatysmal fat. Because these modalities are often

used repetitively, overtreatment of superficial neck anatomy is now an additional problem. Similar to other discussed complications, accurate diagnosis and proper corrective neck surgery have to be done to treat the resultant contour irregularities. Commonly, there is the added problem of inadequate supraplatysmal fat. In these circumstances, microfat injection may be necessary as a secondary procedure to restore natural anatomy.

SUMMARY

Whether attempting to create or restore, a youthful and attractive neck is the goal in plastic surgery, but untoward outcomes can occur. Unsatisfactory results can be caused by unavoidable complications as well as errors in design and execution of procedures. Failures in diagnosis can lead to inaccurate treatment and inadequate results. Native anatomy creates regions of easy access, such as the subcutaneous medial neck and preplatysma muscle, which can lead to issues of overcorrection, whereas regions of difficult access, such as the lateral neck and subplatysma muscle, can lead to problems from undercorrection. Although past discussion of untoward outcomes was restricted to surgical interventions, minimally invasive techniques have now created a new list of issues that need to be addressed.

Because untoward outcomes can occur, understanding their causes, preventing those that are preventable, and accurately diagnosing and treating the issues that occur should be part of every surgeon's skills. This requirement will ensure that ultimately the goal of either creating or restoring a youthful and attractive neck is attained.

REFERENCES

1. Ellenbogen R, Karlin JV. Visual criteria for success in restoring the youthful neck. Plast Reconstr Surg 1980;66(6):826–37.
2. O'Daniel TG. Understanding deep neck anatomy and its clinical relevance. Clin Plast Surg 2018; 45(4):447–54.
3. Mustoe TA, Rawlani V, Zimmerman H. Modified deep plane rhytidectomy with a lateral approach to the neck: an alternative to submental incision and dissection. Plast Reconstr Surg 2011;127(1):357–70.
4. Gordon N, Adam S. Deep plane facelifting for facial rejuvenation. Facial Plast Surg 2014;30(4):394–404.
5. Gonzalez R. The LOPP-lateral overlapping plication of the platysma: an effective neck lift without submental incision. Clin Plast Surg 2014;41(1):65–72.
6. Pelle-Ceravolo M, Angelini M, Silvi E. Treatment of anterior neck aging without a submental approach: lateral skin-platysma displacement, a new and proven technique for platysma bands and skin laxity. Plast Reconstr Surg 2017;139(2):308–21.
7. Marten TJ. High SMAS facelift: combined single flap lifting of the jawline, cheek, and midface. Clin Plast Surg 2008;35(4):569–603. vi-vii.
8. Feldman JJ. Neck lift. St Louis (MO): Quality Medical Pub.; 2006.
9. Gordon NA, Adam SI. The deep-plane approach to neck rejuvenation. Facial Plast Surg Clin North Am 2014;22(2):269–84.
10. Lawrence WT, Plastic Surgery Educational Foundation Data Committee. Nonsurgical face lift. Plast Reconstr Surg 2006;118(2):541–5.
11. Gupta V, Winocour J, Shi H, et al. Preoperative risk factors and complication rates in facelift: analysis of 11,300 patients. Aesthet Surg J 2016;36(1):1–13.
12. O'Daniel TG, Shanahan PT. Dexmedetomidine: a new alpha-agonist anesthetic agent for facial rejuvenation surgery. Aesthet Surg J 2006;26(1):35–40.
13. Auersvald A, Auersvald LA. Hemostatic net in rhytidoplasty: an efficient and safe method for preventing hematoma in 405 consecutive patients. Aesthetic Plast Surg 2014;38(1):1–9.
14. O'Daniel TG, Auersvald A, Auersvald LA. Hemostatic net in facelift surgery. Der MKG-Chirurg 2019; 12(2):78–85.
15. LeRoy JL Jr, Rees TD, Nolan WB 3rd. Infections requiring hospital readmission following face lift surgery: incidence, treatment, and sequelae. Plast Reconstr Surg 1994;93(3):533–6.
16. Van Vliet M, Chai C, Demas C. A prospective look at intraoperative body temperature and various patient demographics and how these relate to postoperative wound infections and other complications. Plast Reconstr Surg 2010;125(2):80e–1e.
17. Moody BR, McCarthy JE, Linder J, et al. Enhanced cosmetic outcome with running horizontal mattress sutures. Dermatol Surg 2005;31(10):1313–6.
18. Del Toro D, Dedhia R, Tollefson TT. Advances in scar management: prevention and management of hypertrophic scars and keloids. Curr Opin Otolaryngol Head Neck Surg 2016;24(4):322–9.
19. Khansa I, Harrison B, Janis JE. Evidence-based scar management: how to improve results with technique and technology. Plast Reconstr Surg 2016; 138(3 Suppl):165S–78S.
20. Gordon NA, Gentile RD. Complications and sequelae of rejuvenation surgery of the neck. In: Gentile RD, editor. Neck rejuvenation. New York: Thieme; 2011. p. 137–45.
21. Ellenbogen R. Pseudo-paralysis of the mandibular branch of the facial nerve after platysmal face-lift operation. Plast Reconstr Surg 1979;63(3):364–8.
22. Daane SP, Owsley JQ. Incidence of cervical branch injury with "marginal mandibular nerve pseudo-paralysis" in patients undergoing face lift. Plast Reconstr Surg 2003;111(7):2414–8.
23. Marten T, Elyassnia D. Management of the platysma in neck lift. Clin Plast Surg 2018;45(4):555–70.
24. Pelle-Ceravolo M, Angelini M, Silvi E. Complete platysma transection in neck rejuvenation: a critical appraisal. Plast Reconstr Surg 2016;138(4):781–91.
25. Mendelson BC, Tutino R. Submandibular gland reduction in aesthetic surgery of the neck: review of 112 consecutive cases. Plast Reconstr Surg 2015;136(3):463–71.
26. Auersvald A, Auersvald LA. Management of the submandibular gland in neck lifts: indications, techniques, pearls, and pitfalls. Clin Plast Surg 2018;45(4):507–25.
27. Bond L, Lee TJ, O'Daniel TG. Strategies for submandibular gland management in rhytidectomy. Clin Surg 2017;2(1446):1–4.
28. ASAPS. Cosmetic surgery National Data Bank statistics, 2017. Available at: https://www.surgery.org/sites/default/files/ASAPS-Stats2017.pdf. Accessed February 12, 2019.

Filler-Associated Vision Loss

Ann Q. Tran, MD, Patrick Staropoli, MD, Andrew J. Rong, MD, Wendy W. Lee, MD, MS*

KEYWORDS

• Filler complications • Central retinal artery occlusion • Vascular obstruction

KEY POINTS

• Soft tissue filler injections have rare and devastating complications, such as permanent vision loss.
• Early recognition of vision loss associated with soft tissue fillers is essential, especially in cases of severe postinjection pain. If vascular occlusion causing vision loss is suspected, referral to ophthalmology should occur immediately.
• With appropriate knowledge of facial anatomy and specific filler characteristics, soft tissue fillers can be injected safely by following tips, such as injecting perpendicular to vessels, avoiding large boluses or excessive injection force, and injecting slowly.
• Potential treatment options of an ophthalmic vascular occlusive event include ocular massage, anterior chamber paracentesis, hyperbaric oxygen, and retrobulbar hyaluronidase injection.

INTRODUCTION

The use of soft tissue fillers continues to gain in popularity, and remains in the top 5 minimally invasive cosmetic procedures with more than 2.69 million performed in 2017.[1] They work to enhance appearance by counteracting volume loss in the aging face. Injected dermal fillers are composed of collagen, hyaluronic acid, polylactic acid, calcium hydroxyapatite, polymethylmetha-crylate, and autologous fat. Complications vary from mild and self-limiting (ecchymosis, swelling, erythema) to more moderate adverse events (over-correction, undercorrection, superficial injection resulting in filler visibility, Tyndall effect, and granuloma formation) and more severe consequences (vision loss, skin necrosis, and anaphylaxis).[2] More than 1700 adverse events were reported between 2014 and 2016 with soft tissue filler injections, of which 8 cases were associated with blindness, a rare but devastating event.[2] Blindness from iatrogenic vascular occlusion is a devastating consequence, often leading to irreversible vision loss and skin necrosis. This article reviews vision loss associated with soft tissue filler injections and appropriate treatment regimens and techniques to avoid intravascular injection.

VASCULAR ANATOMY AND MECHANISM OF VISION LOSS

The vascular supply of the face is highly variable and anastomotic, making it a challenge to comfortably delineate "safe zones" for injection (**Fig. 1**). The blood supply to the orbit begins with the ophthalmic artery, the first branch of the internal carotid and has a limited number of variations and anastomoses.[3,4] The ophthalmic artery then gives off the lacrimal, 2 long ciliary, central retinal, approximately 20 short posterior ciliary, supraorbital, and supratrochlear arteries among others. The central retinal artery enters the dural sheath of the optic nerve approximately 13 mm behind the globe and supplies the inner portion of the retina. The short posterior ciliary arteries supply the choroid and outer retina, with a watershed area at the level of the inner nuclear layer, commonly affected in central retinal artery

Disclosure Statement: Research support from the NIH Center Core Grant P30EY014801.
Bascom Palmer Eye Institute, University of Miami Miller School of Medicine, Miami, FL, USA
* Corresponding author. Bascom Palmer Eye Institute, 900 Northwest 17th Street, Miami, FL, 33136.
E-mail address: WLee@med.miami.edu

Facial Plast Surg Clin N Am 27 (2019) 557–564
https://doi.org/10.1016/j.fsc.2019.07.010

facialplastic.theclinics.com

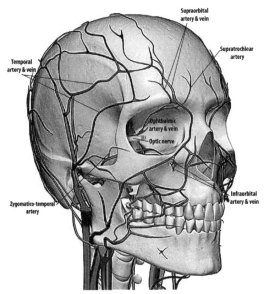

Supraorbital
artery & vein

Supratrochlear
artery

Temporal
artery & vein

Ophthalmic
artery & vein

Optic nerve

Infraorbital
artery & vein

Zygomatico-temporal
artery

Fig. 1. Schematic diagram of the vasculature of the face.

occlusions. Approximately 20% of the population has a cilioretinal artery branch off the short posterior ciliary artery providing alternate perfusion between the macula and the optic nerve.[5]

Occlusion along any part of the vascular supply can cause vision loss. Central retinal artery occlusions tend to cause diffuse inner retinal edema with a cherry red spot on fundoscopic examination. Irreparable damage has been shown to occur in as little as 105 minutes of occlusion.[6,7] Other patterns of ischemia exist: patients with cilioretinal artery sparing can have preserved central vision in the context of a central retinal artery occlusion. In rare cases of cilioretinal artery sparing central retinal artery occlusion, the blood supply to the macula can be preserved with an excellent visual outcome.[8] Ophthalmic artery occlusion results in more devastating consequences of nonperfusion of the entire retina and choroid, whereas branch retinal artery occlusions can vary depending on the area involved. Occlusion of the posterior ciliary arteries can produce variable choroidal and outer retinal ischemia.

Vascular occlusion is thought to occur through a retrograde mechanism in which facial vasculature is infiltrated by a small particle.[3] The force of injection overcomes the systolic blood pressure, and the embolus is pushed backward via anastomoses into the ophthalmic artery. After the injection, systolic pressure can then push the embolus distally into the central retinal artery or other branches of the ophthalmic artery. If the force of the injection is high enough, the embolus could enter the internal carotid artery or anterior,

middle, or posterior cerebral arteries to cause a cerebral infarction.[3] In addition, understanding the properties of soft tissue fillers is important, as their particle size contributes to their ability to occlude vessels. The gel size particle of hyaluronic acid of Restylane-L is approximately 400 μm, which in theory is large enough to block the central retinal artery (160 μm in diameter), compared with the larger ophthalmic artery, which measures 2 mm in greatest diameter.[9]

Understanding the facial anatomy serves as the key to preventing devastating complications.[10–13] The glabella region is generally regarded as a high-risk injection site because the supratrochlear and supraorbital arteries are direct branches off the ophthalmic artery. The supratrochlear artery exits through a foramen at the orbital rim, approximately 1.7 cm from midline, whereas the supraorbital bundle is approximately 2.7 cm from midline.[14] Unfortunately, this corresponds to muscle creases caused by contraction of the glabellar complex and so are often targets for filling. Contraction of these muscles can cause 3 creases: the midline, corrugator, and supraorbital creases. Cadaveric studies have shown that the supratrochlear artery is situated within the corrugator crease and the supraorbital artery is situated within the supraorbital crease. The supraorbital and supratrochlear artery supply the frontalis muscle, coursing subcutaneously 15 to 25 mm above the supraorbital rim.

The temporal region is composed of skin, subcutaneous fat, temporoparietal fascia, and superficial and deep temporal fascia separated by an avascular plane of loose areolar tissue, temporal muscle, periosteum, and bone.[15] Typically, injections are performed with a needle deep on the periosteum or a cannula more superficially in the loose areolar tissue plane. Blood is supplied to this area via the external carotid artery (ECA). The ECA then branches into the maxillary artery, becoming the anterior and posterior deep temporal arteries. Meanwhile, the superficial temporal artery branches directly from the external carotid near the mandible, then travels superiorly 1 cm in front of the ear before turning anteriorly and traversing the zygomatic arch, at which point it is called the frontal branch of the superficial temporal artery.[10–13] This vessel travels within the superficial temporal fascia and is at risk, especially when performing superficial injections.

The superficial temporal artery may anastomose with the supratrochlear or supraorbital artery within the frontalis muscle, providing a retrograde path to the ophthalmic.[10–13] Occasionally, the ophthalmic artery itself arises from the middle meningeal artery, which is a branch of the ECA, providing an even more direct route from superficial temporal artery to the ophthalmic artery. Moreover, the zygomatic-orbital artery, a branch of the superficial temporal artery, occasionally anastomoses with a branch of the ophthalmic.[4]

The infraorbital foramen contains the infraorbital artery. It is located approximately 40% of the distance between the medial and lateral canthi (approximately the medial limbus) up to 11 mm below the infraorbital rim (just less than 1 finger-breadth).[10–13] The second branch of the ECA is the internal maxillary artery. This artery branches into the infraorbital artery, which eventually anastomoses with branches of the supraorbital and supratrochlear vessels. The infraorbital artery lies deep to the levator labii superioris muscle and superficial to the levator anguli oris muscle.

In the nasolabial region, anastomosis of the dorsal nasal artery, angular artery, and lateral nasal artery from the facial artery create a path back to the ophthalmic artery.[10–13] The third branch of the external carotid is the facial artery. It originates at the mandible, transverses medially, gives off the inferior and superior labial arteries, then turns upward along the nasal wall as the angular artery. It runs approximately 5 mm medial to the medial canthal vertical line. The angular artery anastomoses with the dorsal nasal artery, which arises from the ophthalmic artery, pierces through the upper eyelid, and descends along the side of the nose. The dorsal nasal artery is approximately 5 mm above the medial canthal horizontal line. The superior labial artery runs 4.5 mm deep along the upper lip between the oral mucosa and the orbicularis oris muscle. The inferior labial artery originates as the labiomental artery once the facial artery enters the oral vestibule between the platysma and the buccinator muscles.

Anastomoses observed in the terminal branches of the ophthalmic artery seen in cadavers and ultrasound previously help elucidate the anatomic explanation of retrograde travel.[16–18] Looking at an in vivo study with rabbits, methylene blue was injected into the facial artery and the eye was observed for accumulation of dye to look for possible retrograde flow to the retina.[19] Retrograde flow was noted in 1 of 20 rabbits, supporting the theory that filler could enter vessels by direct inoculation or through sites of damage from previous injections. However, systolic blood pressure and dissipation of injection pressure over numerous vascular branches makes it a rare occurrence for emboli to travel retrograde. The complex anastomosis in the orbit and the risk of arterial wall perforations from needles or cannulas are all variables that can cause vision loss from retrograde flow of soft tissue filler.[20]

TYPES OF OCULAR COMPLICATIONS
Ophthalmic, Central Retinal Artery, and Branched Retinal Artery Occlusions

Most cases of soft tissue filler injections result in blindness from retinal artery occlusion (**Fig. 2**). Complications of blindness and vascular compromise with dermal necrosis have been reported with a variety of products in various injection locations.[2] The first reported case of cosmetic facial filler causing a retinal artery occlusion occurred in 1988, and with each passing year, a growing number of cases are reported in the literature.[21]

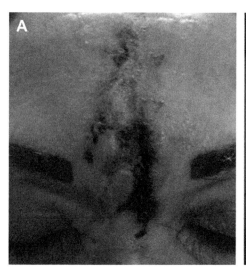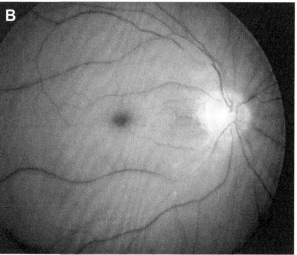

Fig. 2. (A) Skin necrosis following soft tissue filler in the glabellar area. (B) Subsequent central retinal artery occlusion.

Facial injection of soft tissue filler places a patient at risk of iatrogenic vascular occlusion, given the rich anastomosis of the face.

In one of the largest case series of 12 patients with iatrogenic vascular occlusion, ophthalmic artery occlusion (7 cases), branched retinal artery occlusion (3 cases), and central retinal artery occlusion (2 cases) were reported.[22] These cases had injections with autologous fat (7 cases), hyaluronic acid (4 cases), or collagen (1 case); the sites of injection included the glabellar region (7 cases), nasolabial folds (4 cases), or both (1 case). All patients had immediate vision loss, which was most severe in those injected with autologous fat and in those with ophthalmic artery occlusions. Vision was extremely poor from no light perception (7 cases), bare light perception (1 case), or count fingers vision (1 case). Indications of poorer visual prognosis included ocular pain and attenuated choroidal vascularity on optical coherence tomography retinal imaging.

As elucidated earlier when discussing the anatomy of the blood supply, the clinical manifestation depends at the level of vascular occlusion. Iatrogenic ophthalmic artery occlusions have the worst prognosis, with no recoverable vision. As the ophthalmic artery serves as one of the main blood supplies to the orbit and the occlusion occurs proximal to the central retinal artery, both severe vision loss and other ocular findings are typically seen. Ophthalmoplegia, ptosis, and pain all occur due to ischemia of the choroid, levator palpebrae muscle, and ocular muscles supplied by the ophthalmic artery. The severity of vision loss from central retinal artery and branch retinal artery depend on the location and other anastomosis, such as the presence of a cilioretinal artery blood supply to the macula. If the blood supply to the optic nerve is severely compromised, an anterior or posterior ischemic optic neuropathy can occur.[23,24] In rare cases, bilateral blindness with multiple emboli affecting various layers of the retina may occur.[25]

Other Retinal Presentations

Paracentral acute middle maculopathy associated with retinal occlusion after soft tissue filler has been described in 2 cases in which intermediate and deep capillary plexus ischemia occurs.[26,27] Diagnosis is made on optical coherence tomography imaging where retinal hyperreflective whitening occurs on the inner superotemporal macula. Purtscher-like retinopathy can occur in conjunction with paracentral acute middle maculopathy with areas of retinal hemorrhage. In one case, after an oral dose of prednisone and monitoring 4 months later, the hemorrhage resolved and the vision recovered to baseline.[27] The small size of the soft tissue filler has the ability to pass downstream in arterioles and precapillary vessels leading to selective infarction. These cases still result in vision loss, but may have more preserved function compared with ophthalmic and central retinal artery occlusions.

Ocular Ischemic Syndrome

Profound cases of orbital and ocular ischemia can manifest with hypotony, corneal edema, and ophthalmoplegia. A patient injected with 0.8 mL of hyaluronic acid in the dorsum of the nose developed light perception vision with persistent hypotony, complete ophthalmoplegia, a retinal detachment, and skin necrosis. The decision was made to treat the ocular inflammation with high-dose intravenous methylprednisolone 1 g for 3 days and tapered to oral prednisone with concurrent use of aspirin; however, the vision was not regained.[28] In a case of hyaluronic acid injected to the temples and dorsum of the nose, the patient developed no light perception vision, with worsening proptosis, ophthalmoplegia, anterior segment ischemia with hypotony, a hypopyon, and cilioretinal artery occlusion. A retrobulbar injection of 1200 U of hyaluronidase into the orbital apex aided in regaining some orbital function improvement, but the vision was unrecoverable.[29]

Ischemic Oculomotor Palsy

Similar to ocular ischemic syndrome, ophthalmoplegia can occur after secondary vascular occlusion.[30] Some subtle cases may present only with symptoms of diplopia with corresponding imaging highlighting nonspecific orbital inflammation without evidence of emboli.[31] Unlike vision loss, ocular movement can regain some function with treatment. In a patient who received subcutaneous hyaluronidase in the area of skin necrosis, systemic steroids, vasodilation, and lower-level therapy, the ophthalmoplegia induced from soft tissue filler recovered nearly to completion. In many cases associated with ptosis and ophthalmoplegia, follow-up 6 months later showed promising improvement.[32] In more severe cases, ophthalmoplegia may not recover.[33]

Cerebral Infarction

Filler emboli injected into the branches of the ophthalmic artery have the ability to cause retrograde pulsion into the internal carotid artery and retinal cerebral circulation. Combined brain infarction with embolism in the anterior cerebral artery, middle cerebral artery, and circle of Willis have all been described after soft tissue filler injections.[22,33–35] A trial of intravenous and oral steroids did not help regain vision.[34] Neuro-imaging should be considered in filler-related vascular occlusive events and treated similar to an acute ischemic stroke.

TREATMENT OPTIONS

Prompt evaluation and referral to ophthalmology should be performed for patients with vision loss associated with soft tissue dermal fillers. As soon as ocular discomfort is noted, further injection of soft tissue filler should be stopped. In the office, a quick visual acuity test, confrontational visual fields, and pupil examination can be performed by the health care provider. It is advisable to have a vision screening card and a penlight available in the office. Vision checks should be performed with one eye completely occluded for accuracy. Although no reliable treatment exists for iatrogenic retinal embolism; theoretically lowering the intraocular pressure to dislodge the embolus and deliver increased retinal perfusion may be attempted. Reducing the timing of the ischemic period may increase the likelihood of residual function. After 90 minutes, irreversible retinal ischemia and necrosis occur.[6,7,36,37]

Historical treatment stems from conservative treatments of central retinal artery occlusions from noniatrogenic causes.[38] The patient can be laid supine, ocular digital massage can be performed, acetazolamide (500 mg oral or intravenous) or 20% Mannitol solution in a 250-mL normal saline solution can be given, or topical aqueous suppression may be applied. The mechanical pressure of the ocular massage in theory could help dislodge the embolus and lower intraocular pressure, although cases in which this has been attempted have been ineffective.[22,39–42] Acetazolamide can lead to reduced intraocular pressure and increase in retinal blood flow, but again without much success in regaining vision. Anterior chamber paracentesis performed with a 30 gauge 1/2 inch needle can allow for egress of aqueous fluid and corresponding decrease in intraocular pressure; however, this has not had promising results.[39]

In ophthalmologic studies of central retinal artery occlusions treated within 20 hours of onset with a visual acuity worse than 20/60, the use of topical beta blocker (timolol 0.5%), intravenous injection of 500 mg acetazolamide, and ocular massage resulted in visual improvement in 60% of patients.[43] None of these patients were reported to be no light perception. Other experimental treatments for central retinal artery occlusions have been attempted, but are currently not recommended as standard of care. The use of local intra-arterial fibrinolysis with a maximum of 50 mg tPA within 20 hours of the development of a central retinal artery occlusion did not show any significant differences compared with treatment with conservative therapy. One-third of these patients additionally had complaints of headache to more severe complications, such as vascular hematoma, intracranial hemorrhage, and permanent hemiparesis.[43]

The role of hyperbaric oxygen leads to dilation of the retinal arterioles and a high amount of oxygen delivered to ischemic tissues.[44,45] One patient with a combined central retinal vein and cilioretinal artery occlusion who underwent 14 days of hyperbaric treatment (2 hours per day), regained vision from 20/200 to 20/20. However, this patient did not have an iatrogenic cause of the occlusive event. Patients with ophthalmic artery obstruction after hyaluronic acid treated with hyperbaric oxygen have not been shown to have improved visual outcomes.[46,47]

Hyaluronidase is an endogenous enzyme that can hydrolyze and depolymerize hyaluronic acid fillers.[48] Hyaluronidase should be available in all offices that perform soft tissue injections, as immediate reversal of filler application can be given at any early sign of adverse events. In animal models, retrobulbar injection of hyaluronidase after an ophthalmic artery occlusive episode with hyaluronic acid gel was unable to recover or restore visual function.[49] Hyaluronidase may have greatest effectivity at the immediate vessel it is injected at because it may penetrate through the vessel walls, but may not be able to reach the retinal circulation to restore perfusion,[50] given that the central retinal artery runs through the center of the optic nerve, which is likely impenetrable to the enzyme. Case reports with retrobulbar hyaluronidase to restore vision have been unsuccessful.[33,51] In one case, reported visual improvement occurred after injection of 450 IU of retrobulbar hyaluronidase; however, there was no ophthalmic examination at the time to determine the etiology of vision loss.[52] The use of interventional radiology for direct intra-arterial injection and intravenous injection of hyaluronidase in animal models have not shown promising results in ability to restore vision.[53]

The use of oral and intravenous corticosteroids may help reduce the inflammatory response from the resulting iatrogenic vascular occlusive event. Similar to the treatment results of traumatic optic neuropathy, corticosteroids provide little return of vision.[54] Notably, there has been utility in its use in patients with anterior segment and orbital ischemia with ophthalmoplegia, as these patients had improvement of anterior chamber inflammation, orbital swelling, and extraocular motility.[29–31]

PREVENTION TECHNIQUES

The literature describes various preventive strategies. Local anesthesia with epinephrine constricts arteries, reducing risk of cannulation. Aspiration always should be performed before injection to rule out intravascular cannulation, but it is important not to get a false sense of security if a flash of blood is not seen, as very small movements of the syringe can result in a different position of the needle or cannula. Limit injected filler volume with each pass and inject slowly to decrease ejection pressure.[3] Avoiding the corrugator and supraorbital creases is paramount, as these vessels are in closest proximity to the ophthalmic artery, and digital pressure should be used to occlude these creases along the rim to prevent backflow.[10] An anterograde/retrograde injection technique, keeping the needle in constant motion while injecting in small increments, should be used. Low-pressure injection is key if significant resistance is encountered, as it could be intravascular pressure, a fibrous septum, or a clogged needle. In this case, repositioning and replacing the needle should be attempted. Many of the techniques described in the following paragraphs are based on the author's personal experience.

Some argue that use of a cannula may be safer; however, in cadaver studies, cannulas can still penetrate the artery, particularly when inserted perpendicularly into an artery that is fixed by a fibrous septum, stretched in a tortuous position, or at a bifurcation.[20] A larger cannula (22G or 25G) with parallel insertion may decrease the risk of penetration, as the cannula should brush arteries aside. Conversely, needles can penetrate an artery at any angle and should be inserted perpendicularly to decrease the chance they come into contact with a vessel. Smaller-gauge needles can be considered, but keep in mind that if the needle is smaller than the vessel, penetration can occur.

Specific considerations when injecting temporally include palpating, marking, and avoiding the superficial temporal artery. Injecting on the periosteum, deep to the temporoparietal fascia, or subcutaneously has been described.[15] These recommendations also suggest hyaluronic acid–based fillers in this tissue plane as opposed to previous recommendations for calcium hydroxylapatite or poly-L-lactic acid placed below the temporalis muscle. When injecting on the periosteum, an imaginary "safe" boundary is described consisting of a region superomedially at the temporal fusion line at the tail of brow, inferiorly at a line 1.5 cm above the zygomatic arch (avoiding the middle temporal vein), and posteriorly at the hairline. An alternative methodology of injecting includes 1 cm superior and 1 cm lateral to the tail of the brow.

In the glabellar region, superficial injection is relatively safe because the supraorbital and supratrochlear arteries are located deep, whereas in the upper forehead region, deep injection on the periosteum is advised, as the vessels ascend superficially. In the infraorbital area, deep injections should be placed only lateral to the infraorbital foramen (approximately medial limbus). If filler is needed medially, it can be injected lateral to the foramen then massaged over.

In the nasolabial area, injections in the deep dermis or superficial subcutaneous tissue should be performed in the inferior two-thirds of the nasolabial fold with an anterograde and/or retrograde linear threading technique. The upper third of the nasolabial fold should be injected at the preperiosteal level because the artery is subdermal at this level. Periosteal injection may be safer than in the sub-superficial musculoaponeurotic system plane. Regardless, digital compression of the angular and dorsal nasal arteries is recommended. Injecting 2 to 3 mm above the alar groove helps avoid the lateral nasal artery.

Fortunately, no clinical evidence to date supports blindness following lip augmentation; however, several precautions should still be taken. A safe technique is using a cannula or needle with small injections parallel to the lip margin. Great care should be taken at the medial third segment where the artery courses superficially at the wet–dry junction, particularly in the upper lip. Deep injection around the oral commissure, submucosal injection of the medial and middle segments of the vermilion zone, and submucosal injections within oral mucosa are discouraged because of the high risk of arterial injury.[17]

SUMMARY

Facial soft tissue fillers have the possibility of rare and irreversible ophthalmic complications. Although this minimally invasive cosmetic procedure is considered generally safe, prevention of adverse events requires proper injection technique, early recognition of complications, and prompt treatment. However, most cases end tragically with the inability to regain vision loss.

REFERENCES

1. American Society of Plastics Surgeons. 2017 national clearinghouse of plastic surgery 2018. p. 1–4. Available at: https://www.plasticsurgery.org/news/plastic-surgery-statistics.
2. Rayess HM, Svider PF, Hanba C, et al. A cross-sectional analysis of adverse events and litigation for injectable fillers. JAMA Facial Plast Surg 2018; 20(3):207–14.
3. Li X, Du L, Lu JJ. A novel hypothesis of visual loss secondary to cosmetic facial filler injection. Ann Plast Surg 2015;75(3):258–60.
4. Bertelli E, Regoli M, Bracco S. An update on the variations of the orbital blood supply and hemodynamic. Surg Radiol Anat 2017;39(5):485–96.
5. Justice J Jr, Lehmann RP. Cilioretinal arteries. A study based on review of stereo fundus photographs and fluorescein angiographic findings. Arch Ophthalmol 1976;94(8):1355–8.
6. Hayreh SS, Weingeist TA. Experimental occlusion of the central artery of the retina: IV. Retinal tolerance time to acute ischaemia. Br J Ophthalmol 1980;64:818–25.
7. Hayreh SS, Zimmerman MB, Kimura A, et al. Central retinal artery occlusion. Retinal survival time. Exp Eye Res 2004;78(3):723–36.
8. Doguizi S, Sekeroglu MA, Anayol MA, et al. Central retinal artery occlusion with double cilioretinal artery sparing. Retin Cases Brief Rep 2019;13(1):75–8.
9. Gold MH. Use of hyaluronic acid fillers for the treatment of the aging face. Clin Interv Aging 2007;2(3):369–76.
10. Scheuer JF 3rd, Sieber DA, Pezeshk RA, et al. Facial danger zones: techniques to maximize safety during soft-tissue filler injections. Plast Reconstr Surg 2017;139(5):1103–8.
11. Bentsianov B, Blitzer A. Facial anatomy. Clin Dermatol 2004;22:3–13.
12. Ferneini EM, Hapelas S, Watras J, et al. Surgeon's guide to facial soft tissue filler injections: relevant anatomy and safety considerations. J Oral Maxillofac Surg 2017;75(12):2667.e1-5.
13. Wu S, Pan L, Wu H, et al. Anatomic study of ophthalmic artery embolism following cosmetic injection. J Craniofac Surg 2017;28(6):1578–81.
14. Pessa JE, Rohrich RJ. Facial topography clinical anatomy of the face. St Louis (MO): Quality Medical Publishing Inc; 2012.
15. Breithaupt AD, Jones DH, Braz A, et al. Anatomical basis for safe and effective volumization of the temple. Dermatol Surg 2015;41(Suppl 1):S278–83.
16. Tansatit T, Moon HJ, Apinuntrum P, et al. Verification of embolic channel causing blindness following filler injection. Aesthetic Plast Surg 2015;39:154–61.
17. Tansatit T, Phumyoo T, Jitaree B, et al. Cadaveric assessment of lip injections: locating the serious threats. Aesthetic Plast Surg 2017;41:430–40.
18. Tansatit T, Phumyoo T, Jitaree B, et al. Ultrasound evaluation of arterial anastomosis of the forehead. J Cosmet Dermatol 2018;17:1031–6.
19. Zheng H, Qiu L, Liu Z, et al. Exploring the possibility of a retrograde embolism pathway from the facial artery to the ophthalmic artery system in vivo. Aesthetic Plast Surg 2017;41(5):1222–7.
20. Tansatit T, Apinuntrum PT. A dark side of the cannula injections: how arterial wall perforations and emboli occur. Aesthetic Plast Surg 2017;41:221–7.
21. Shin H, Lemke BN, Stevens TS, et al. Posterior ciliary-artery occlusion after subcutaneous silicone-oil injection. Ann Ophthalmol 1988;20:342–4.
22. Park SW, Woo SJ, Park KH, et al. Iatrogenic retinal artery occlusion caused by cosmetic facial filler injections. Am J Ophthalmol 2012;154(4):653–62.
23. Chen Y, Wang W1, Li J, et al. Fundus artery occlusion caused by cosmetic facial injections. Chin Med J (Engl) 2014;127(8):1434–7.
24. Kim A, Kim SH, Kim HJ, et al. Ophthalmoplegia as a complication of cosmetic facial filler injection. Acta Ophthalmol 2016;94(5):e377–9.
25. Kim YJ, Choi KS. Bilateral blindness after filler injection. Plast Reconstr Surg 2013;131(2):298e–9e.
26. Sridhar J, Shahlaee A, Shieh WS, et al. Paracentral acute middle maculopathy associated with retinal artery occlusion after cosmetic filler injection. Retin Cases Brief Rep 2017;11(Suppl 1):S216–8.
27. Khatibi A. Brazilian booty retinopathy: Purtscher-like retinopathy with paracentral acute middle maculopathy associated with PMMA injection into buttocks. Retin Cases Brief Rep 2018;12(1):17–20.
28. Kim YJ, Kim SS, Song WK, et al. Ocular ischemia with hypotony after injection of hyaluronic acid gel. Ophthalmic Plast Reconstr Surg 2011;27(6):e152–5.
29. Ramesh S, Fiaschetti D, Goldberg RA. Orbital and ocular ischemic syndrome with blindness after facial filler injection. Ophthalmic Plast Reconstr Surg 2018; 34(4):e108–10.
30. Bae IH, Kim MS, Choi H, et al. Ischemic oculomotor nerve palsy due to hyaluronic acid filler injection. J Cosmet Dermatol 2018;17(6):1016–8.
31. Dagi Glass LR, Choi CJ, Lee NG. Orbital complication following calcium hydroxylapatite filler injection. Ophthalmic Plast Reconstr Surg 2017;33(3S Suppl 1):S16–7.
32. Myung Y, Yim S, Jeong JH, et al. The classification and prognosis of periocular complications related to blindness following cosmetic filler injection. Plast Reconstr Surg 2017;140(1):61–4.
33. Kim SN, Byun DS, Park JH, et al. Panophthalmoplegia and vision loss after cosmetic nasal dorsum injection. J Clin Neurosci 2014;21(4):678–80.

34. Ragam A, Agemy SA, Dave SB, et al. Ipsilateral ophthalmic and cerebral infarctions after cosmetic polylactic acid injection into the forehead. J Neuroophthalmol 2017;37(1):77–80.

35. Sellés-Navarro I, Villegas-Pérez MP, Salvador-Silva M, et al. Retinal ganglion cell death after different transient periods of pressure-induced ischemia and survival intervals: a quantitative in vivo study. Invest Ophthalmol Vis Sci 1996;37(10):2002–14.

36. Sellés-Navarro I, Villegas-Pérez MP, Salvador-Silva M, et al. Retinal ganglion cell death after different transient periods of pressure-induced ischemia and survival intervals: a quantitative in vivo study. Invest Ophthalmol Vis Sci 1996;37:2002–14.

37. Roth S, Li B, Rosenbaum PS, et al. Preconditioning provides complete protection against retinal ischemic injury in rats. Invest Ophthalmol Vis Sci 1998;39:775–85.

38. Loh KT, Chua JJ, Lee HM, et al. Prevention and management of vision loss relating to facial filler injections. Singapore Med J 2016;57(8):438–43.

39. Tangsirichaipong A. Blindness after facial contour augmentation with injectable silicone. J Med Assoc Thai 2009;92(Suppl 3):S85–7.

40. Lee DH, Yang HN, Kim JC, et al. Sudden unilateral visual loss and brain infarction after autologous fat injection into nasolabial groove. Br J Ophthalmol 1996;80:1026–7.

41. von Bahr G. Multiple embolisms in the fundus of an eye after an injection in the scalp. Acta Ophthalmol (Copenh) 1963;41:85–91.

42. Ffytche TJ. A rationalization of treatment of central retinal artery occlusion. Trans Ophthalmol Soc U K 1974;94:468–79.

43. Schumacher M, Schmidt D, Jurklies B, et al. Central retinal artery occlusion: local intra-arterial fibrinolysis versus conservative treatment, a multicenter randomized trial. Ophthalmology 2010;117:1367–75.e1.

44. Hwang K. Hyperbaric oxygen therapy to avoid blindness from filler injection. J Craniofac Surg 2016;27(8):2154–5.

45. Celebi AR, Kilavuzoglu AE, Altiparmak UE, et al. Hyperbaric oxygen for the treatment of the rare combination of central retinal vein occlusion and cilioretinal artery occlusion. Diving Hyperb Med 2016;46(1):50–3.

46. Carle MV, Roe R, Novack R, et al. Cosmetic facial fillers and severe vision loss. JAMA Ophthalmol 2014;132(5):637–9.

47. Mori K, Ohta K, Nagano S, et al. A case of ophthalmic artery obstruction following autologous fat injection in the glabellar area (in Japanese). Nippon Ganka Gakkai Zasshi 2007;111:22–5.

48. Bailey SH, Fagien S, Rohrich RJ. Changing role of hyaluronidase in plastic surgery. Plast Reconstr Surg 2014;133:127e–32e.

49. Hwang CJ, Mustak H, Gupta AA, et al. Role of retrobulbar hyaluronidase in filler-associated blindness: evaluation of fundus perfusion and electroretinogram readings in an animal model. Ophthalmic Plast Reconstr Surg 2019;35(1):33–7.

50. DeLorenzi C. Complications of injectable fillers, part 2: vascular complications. Aesthet Surg J 2014;34:584–600.

51. Chestnut C. Restoration of visual loss with retrobulbar hyaluronidase injection after hyaluronic acid filler. Dermatol Surg 2018;44(3):435–7.

52. Zhu G, Sun Z, Liao W, et al. Efficacy of retrobulbar hyaluronidase injection for vision loss resulting from hyaluronic acid filler embolization. Aesthet Surg J 2017;38:12–22.

53. Kim DW, Yoon ES, Ji YH, et al. Vascular complications of hyaluronic acid fillers and the role of hyaluronidase in management. J Plast Reconstr Aesthet Surg 2011;64:1590–5.

54. Guy WM, Soparkar CN, Alford EL, et al. Traumatic optic neuropathy and second optic nerve injuries. JAMA Ophthalmol 2014;132(5):567–71.

Management of Lip Complications

Amar Gupta, MD, Philip J. Miller, MD*

KEYWORDS

- Lip rejuvenation • Injectable fillers • Lip fillers • Nonsurgical lip augmentation
- Lip filler complications

KEY POINTS

- The classification of filler complications to the lips can be divided according to severity (mild, moderate, severe), nature (ischemic complications and nonischemic), or by time of onset (immediate, early, or late).
- Immediate (up to 24 hours after injection) and early (24 hours to 4 weeks after injections) complications of filler injections to the lips include ecchymosis, swelling, infections, herpetic outbreak, nodules, and vascular compromise.
- Late and delayed (greater than 4 weeks after injection) include ecchymosis, swelling, skin discoloration, hyperpigmentation, infection, and nodule formation.
- The late complications are similar to those seen in the immediate and early phase but often represent a more chronic and protracted course, often requiring additional, sometimes more invasive, treatment modalities.

INTRODUCTION

Procedures on the lips have become increasingly common and popularity has grown due to cultural trends and association of lip appearance with both youth and beauty. The number of procedures involving soft tissue fillers has increased from 1.6 million in 2011 to more than 2.4 million in 2015.[1] The growing use of dermal fillers, specifically the use of hyaluronic acid (HA), can be explained by their effectiveness and versatility, as well as their favorable safety profiles.

There has been a surge in the so-called prejuvenation trend, with younger patients wishing to remain youthful and seeking care earlier rather than waiting to turn back the clock on the aging process later in life. In 2018, 72% of facial plastic surgeons saw an increase in cosmetic surgery or injectables in patients younger than age 30 years. This represented a 24% increase in cosmetic surgery or injectables in this age group since 2013 (58% to 72%).[2]

Many patients desire filler injection to the lips to improve the fullness and definition of this anatomic structure. As individuals age, the upper lip lengthens and may develop a thinned appearance. This is important to consider because an aged mouth in the center of an otherwise rejuvenated face looks odd.[3] A long, aging lip is often present and addressing this finding typically requires direct perioral incisions. Fillers into and around the lips are a useful adjunct in these patients. The lip and perioral area is generally not addressed by traditional lifting techniques that place incisions around the ears or under the eyes. Multiple factors contribute to this phenomenon, including the elasticity of the facial soft tissues, the resistance of the nasolabial folds to remote pulling or tightening, and the intimate relation of the perioral skin to the underlying orbicularis

Disclosure Statement: None.
Department of Otolaryngology–Head and Neck Surgery, New York University School of Medicine, 550 First Avenue, NBV 5E5, New York, NY 10016, USA
* Corresponding author.
E-mail address: pjm@gothamplasticsurgeryny.com

Facial Plast Surg Clin N Am 27 (2019) 565–570
https://doi.org/10.1016/j.fsc.2019.07.011

facialplastic.theclinics.com

muscle.[4] These factors all point to the importance of a direct approach to perioral aging and aesthetics. Soft tissue filler for augmentation of the lips and perioral region plays a significant role in rejuvenation of this region. These procedures are associated with significant complications that the surgeon must be aware of.[5]

This article reviews the complications associated with dermal filler injections to the lips and discusses best practices for management of these complications. Evidence-based recommendations for both prevention and treatment of these complications are discussed.

FILLER COMPLICATIONS

The use of soft tissue fillers is becoming increasingly prevalent and is commonly requested by patients who desire fuller lips with more definition. Though filler injections are associated with satisfactory results in many patients, the number of complications is increasing owing to the increased use of these injectable compounds. Fortunately, the incidence of complications is low and most adverse events are mild.[6,7] It is important to note that the proper selection and placement of product can help avoid some complications.[8]

The classification of filler complications can be divided according to severity (mild, moderate, severe), nature (ischemic complications and nonischemic), or by time of onset (early or late).[9,10] Rohrich and colleagues[11] initially proposed a system of classification that suggested that complications should be classified as early (less than 14 days), late (14 days to 1 year), and delayed (more than 1 year) because these time frames correlate well with the potential underlying etiologic factors. Newer classification systems have classified complications as immediate (up to 24 hours after procedure), early onset (24 hours to 4 weeks), and delayed onset (more than 4 weeks).[12] The immediate and early complications are often discussed together.

Immediate and early complications of filler injections to the lips include ecchymosis, swelling, infections, herpetic outbreak, and nodules.

Ecchymosis

Ecchymosis, or bruising, is a common complication of filler injections and is observed more frequently after injection into the immediate submucosal plane, especially when using a fanning or threading technique.[13] The risk of bruising is reduced by slow injection. If bruising appears during the procedure, it can be reduced by compression.[6] The use of blunt cannulas has also become increasingly popular for reducing bruising and

swelling.[14] Cold compress, arnica, aloe vera, and vitamin K creams have all been used to treat bruising after the procedure.[9,15,16] If possible, anticoagulant substances such as nonsteroidal antiinflammatory drug medications (NSAIDs), many herbal or vitamin supplements, and antiplatelet agents should be discontinued for 7 to 10 days before the filler treatment.[6,16–19] It is also advisable to avoid strenuous activity or exercise for 24 hours after the procedure because this helps further reduce the risk of bruising and swelling.[17]

Swelling

Swelling, or edema, that is transient in nature and occurs immediately after the procedure is normal. This may vary in severity and timing based on the specific product used.[9] The lip is among the most commonly affected areas and factors that influence the amount of swelling include injection volume, technique, and patient factors such as dermographism.[16] Preprocedure medications, such as bromelain and arnica, as well as cold compresses have been used in an attempt to prevent swelling after treatment. Management of concerning swelling postprocedure differs based on severity of the condition. For mild swelling, the same agents used preprocedure are recommended. Moderate swelling may require the use of various NSAIDs. Severe swelling may require the use of corticosteroids such as prednisone. The goal is to use the lowest dose and for the shortest time.[12] Dermal fillers are essentially foreign bodies and, in rare cases, patients may develop a hypersensitivity to these compounds. This immune response may be a more acute immunoglobulin E (IgE)-mediated type I hypersensitivity (ie, typically subsides within a few days with oral antihistamines and/or oral steroids) or a delayed type IV hypersensitivity (ie, nonresponsive to antihistamines and requires treatment with hyaluronidase).

Infection

Any procedure that breaks the surface of the skin, including dermal filler injection, carries with it a risk of infection. Acute infections, which present as acute inflammation or abscess formation, are typically due to common skin flora such as *Staphylococcus aureus* or *Streptococcus pyogenes*. Mild forms respond to oral antibiotics and recommendations are for amoxicillin-clavulanic acid or ciprofloxacin for treatment with a course of 14 days.[9,20]

Herpetic Outbreak

Dermal filler injections can lead to reactivation of herpes virus infections and the perioral area accounts for a major anatomic site where herpetic reactivations occur.[9] Injections should be delayed in patients with active herpes lesions. In those with a history of severe cold sores, treatment with an antiviral medication (eg, valacyclovir) is recommended 1 day before and 3 days after filler injection.[16,17]

Nodules

Nodules are some of the most common complications associated with filler injections.[16] Nodules can be classified according to their type (noninflammatory, inflammatory, or infectious), as well as their time of presentation (early, late, or delayed).[11] Early nodules present within days or weeks, are generally painless, and are thought to be the result of suboptimal techniques such as excess filler use, superficial injection, and use of an incorrect product for the indication.[16,21] Early posttreatment nodules may respond to massage. If the nodule is believed to be inflammatory and inflammation is improving, observation may be all that is needed. Noninflammatory nodules are addressed by needle aspiration, minimal stab wound incision with evacuation, and/or hyaluronidase injection.[12]

Late and Delayed Complications

Late and delayed complications of dermal fillers include ecchymosis, swelling, skin discoloration, hyperpigmentation, infection, and nodule formation.

Ecchymosis

Ecchymosis or bruising is usually an early-onset complication but persistent staining may occur in some patients. Vascular lasers such as the pulsed dye laser of potassium titanyl phosphate (KTP) can help speed recovery in these cases.[9,16]

Swelling

Delayed edema may be a result of either an antibody or nonantibody-mediated process. Though antibody-mediated edema typically resolves in the short term, episodes lasting more than 6 weeks may be observed. Edema in these cases should be controlled with the smallest dose of oral corticosteroids that is effective.[9] Additional treatment options that have been proposed include intralesional steroids and immunosuppressive agents.[6] Nonantibody-mediated edema is typically a delayed type IV hypersensitivity reaction that is T cell–mediated. It is characterized by edema, erythema, and induration that usually occurs 1 day after injection but may be seen as late as several weeks after injection and may persist for many months.[22] Antihistamines are not effective in these reactions and the best approach is to remove the filler compound, which is serving as an allergen and is the inciting force for persistent inflammation. Hyaluronidase is recommended for HA fillers, whereas other filler materials may require treatment with steroids until the material resorbs, laser treatment, and/or extrusion. Excision may be required in rare circumstances as a last resort[23] (Fig. 1).

Skin Discoloration

Multiple types of skin discoloration have been observed in the late period, including neovascularization, hyperpigmentation, and the Tyndall effect. Neovascularization refers to the formation of new capillaries, arterioles, and venules that occur as a result of the tissue trauma caused by filler injection. These new vessels should fade within 3 to 12 months without further treatment, but laser treatment has been shown to be effective in recalcitrant cases.[12] Hyperpigmentation is not uncommon after dermal filler injection, especially in patients with Fitzpatrick skin types IV to VI.[24,25] This complication is typically more commonly seen at cutaneous sites rather than within the lips themselves. The first-line therapeutic approach in these cases is with bleaching agents such as topical 4% to 8% hydroquinone and tretinoin (Retin-A) combined with a daily broad-spectrum sunscreen.[12] Chemical peels, intense pulsed light, pulsed dye laser, and fractional laser have also been used to address this complication.[9] The Tyndall effect refers to a bluish hue that becomes apparent when particulate HA fillers are inappropriately injected too superficially.[26] This can last for a very long period of time and

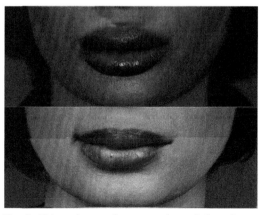

Fig. 1. This patient underwent poly methyl methacrylate (Artefill) injection to the lip elsewhere and was unsatisfied with the aesthetic outcome. Surgical correction was carried out, consisting of upper and lower lip reduction: preoperative (*top*) and postoperative (*bottom*).

even persist for years if not adequately treated. Hyaluronidase is the recommended initial treatment recommendation. If this does not adequately address the dyspigmentation, a small-gauge needle or surgical scalpel can be used to express the superficially placed filler as long as 12 months after initial injection.[27,28]

Infection

Delayed-onset and chronic infections develop 2 or more weeks after injection, tend to affect a more generalized area, and may involve atypical organisms such as *Escherichia coli* or mycobacteria. These infections are difficult to diagnose and can lead to a chronic inflammatory response. A clinical assessment is paramount to assess whether the appropriate treatment is antibiotics or corticosteroids.[12] A bacterial culture may be a helpful adjunct in this situation. Though abscess formation is rare, it may occur in the late period and first-line therapy is drainage and antibiotics.[29] Of note, low-grade infections have been linked to the development of many delayed-onset complications, including foreign body granulomas as a result of biofilm formation.[20]

Nodules

Nodules and lumps, as previously noted, are common complications resulting from the use of dermal fillers in the lips. Nodules, in the late phase, are also characterized as inflammatory and noninflammatory in nature. Delayed onset nodules (from 4 weeks to 1 year or even longer) are usually inflammatory (ie, immune response to filler material) and/or related to infection (eg, biofilm).[30,31] Biofilms consist of densely packed communities of bacteria that surround themselves with the polymers they secrete. Bacteria in biofilms have been detected in biopsies despite negative cultures.[32] Molecular techniques such as polymerase chain reaction and fluorescence in situ hybridization may thus be useful to detect bacteria in these delayed-onset nodules in which biofilm formation is suspected.[30] As biofilms progress, they become more resistant to antibiotics and growth on culture. The treatment is removal of the foreign material, which can consist of hyaluronidase, which should not be used in the presence of an active infection or cellulitis because it can facilitate spread of infection into adjacent tissues.[33] Additional strategies for treating biofilms include low doses of triamcinolone mixed with 5-fluorouracil (5-FU) injected at regular intervals until resolution.[16] More recent evidence has shown efficacy of human platelet-rich plasma to help in management of bacterial biofilms.[34,35] Antibiotics recommended in these cases include prolonged courses of ciprofloxacin or minocycline.[17]

It is extremely difficult to distinguish inflammation secondary to bacterial biofilm from a low-grade hypersensitivity reaction. These hypersensitivity reactions can lead to foreign-body granuloma formation. The incidence of these granulomas is extremely rare (0.01%–1%) and they typically appear after a latent period, which can be several months to years after the injection.[36,37] These reactions can be treated with hyaluronidase dosed at 150 U/mL. Granulomas may respond to oral or intralesional steroids, and addition of 5-FU to intralesional corticosteroids may be a useful adjunct. Surgical excision is the treatment of choice if other therapies repeatedly fail[16,17] (**Fig. 2**).

SURGICAL CORRECTION

The senior author's surgical solution for nodular formation or hypertrophy of the lips due to prior permanent filler involves the following maneuvers:

- With the patient in front of the mirror, and with their lips relaxed, a marking pen is used to draw a line where the upper and lower lip touch each other. This is accomplished with a simple glide of a marking pen across the

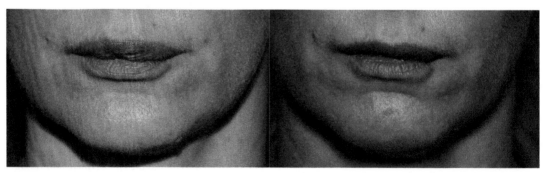

Fig. 2. This patient underwent prior silicone injections to the lip with resulting irregularity and nodularity, notably in the upper lip. Surgical correction was required, consisting of upper lip reduction: preoperative (*left*) and postoperative (*right*).

lips that will paint the upper and lower lip simultaneously. The lips are then patted dry to remove all excess ink.

- The patient is then asked to approximate the size of both upper and lower lips as they would like it to look postoperatively. This is marked in a similar fashion.
- The distance (central height of the drawn fusiform) between the 2 lines is then transferred to just posterior to the original line drawn, adding 10% to 15% additional height owing to anticipated stretching and elasticity of the mucosa. A fusiform incision is drawn starting approximately 3 mm from the oral commissure, encompassing the entire length of the lip to the contralateral side, with care not to involve the oral commissure as well. Adjustment of the length of the fusiform incision is based on the width of the lip deformity. For focal irregularities, the incision need not extend the entire lip length.
- Before injection, the patient is reminded that, due to scarring, inflation of the lip with injection may disproportionately enlarge 1 region more than another, which will persist immediately postoperatively, creating what appears to be asymmetry. The patient is assured that the lines that were drawn preinjection demonstrate what will be removed and thus any irregularities immediately postoperatively are due to the asymmetry of the injection not of the excision and will resolve within the week. The entire region is infiltrated with 1% lidocaine, 1/8% bupivacaine hydrochloride (Marcaine), and 1: 100,000 epinephrine. The patient is then prepped and draped.
- An assistant retracts both oral commissures, placing lateral tension bilaterally. A number 15 blade incises the mucosa to the level of the underlying muscle fascia. The most anterior incision is typically just posterior to the wet–dry junction. The tissue to be excised is grasped with Adson-Brown forceps and serrated scissors are used to remove the tissue in a uniform plane while gliding on top of the underlying muscle and avoiding the arterial supply.
- Most important, do not attempt to intentionally and independently resect the permanent material. This has resulted in multiple lip irregularities, asymmetries, and abnormalities. The permanent filler is treated as if this is a simple lip reduction and as if there were no filler responsible for the size of the lip. In the senior author's experience, this has not resulted in breakdown of the wound nor long-term irregularities.

- Hemostasis is maintained with bipolar cautery.
- The incision is then reapproximated centrally with a buried 4-0 chromic suture with its tail left long and then run locked toward the commissure. An additional suture, buried, begins at the contralateral commissure toward the midline and tied to the original buried suture.

Important insights include

- Careful discussion must be had to distinguish between the patient's desire to decrease the anterior posterior projection of the lip versus the vertical height of the red lip.
- If an anterior to posterior deprojection is required, this can be accomplished with an incision followed by debulking of the underlying soft tissue or filler without excision of mucosa, understanding the limitation of the deprojection based on the placement of the teeth and gums.
- Patients are advised that they will proceed through a period of numbness and a feeling of contracture for several weeks that will resolve typically at 3 months.

A video reference is available at https://youtu.be/PeS8xdxujv8.

SUMMARY

Recently, the use of soft tissue fillers, especially those with HA formulations, has significantly increased. A thorough understanding of the complications and sequelae of this treatment is paramount to safe and effective injection practices and postprocedure management. This article outlined the nonvascular complications associated with soft tissue filler injections to the lips, including those that are immediate and early, as well as those that present in a late or delayed fashion. Evidence-based recommendations both for prevention and treatment of these complications were discussed.

REFERENCES

1. American SOCIETY of Plastic Surgeons: 2014 Plastic surgery statistics report. Available at: http://www.plasticsurgery.org/Documents/news-resources/statistics/2014-statistics/plasticsurgery- statistics-full-report.pdf.
2. American Academy of Facial Plastic and Reconstructive Surgery: 2018 Annual Survey. Available at: https://www.aafprs.org/media/stats_polls/m_stats.html.
3. Foad N. Art of aesthetic surgery. St Louis (MO): Thieme; 2010.
4. Austin H, Weston G. Rejuvenation of the aging mouth. Clin Plast Surg 1992;19:511–24.

5. Austin H. The lip lift. Plast Reconstr Surg 1986;77: 990–4.

6. De Boulle K, Heydenrych I. Patient factors influencing dermal filler complications: prevention, assessment, and treatment. Clin Cosmet Investig Dermatol 2015;8:205–14.

7. Ferneini EM, Ferneini AM. An overview of vascular adverse events associated with facial soft tissue fillers: recognition, prevention, and treatment. J Oral Maxillofac Surg 2016;74(8):1630–6.

8. Sundaram H, Cassuto D. Biophysical characteristics of hyaluronic acid soft-tissue fillers and their relevance to aesthetic applications. Plast Reconstr Surg 2013;132(4 Suppl 2):5S–21S.

9. Funt D, Pavicic T. Dermal fillers in aesthetics: an overview of adverse events and treatment approaches. Plast Surg Nurs 2015;35:13–32.

10. Wagner RD, Fakhro A, Cox JA, et al. Etiology, prevention, and management of infectious complications of dermal fillers. Semin Plast Surg 2016;30(2): 83–6.

11. Rohrich RJ, Nguyen AT, Kenkel JM. Lexicon for soft tissue implants. Dermatol Surg 2009;35(Suppl 2): 1605–11.

12. Urdiales-gálvez F, Delgado NE, Figueiredo V, et al. Treatment of soft tissue filler complications: expert consensus recommendations. Aesthetic Plast Surg 2018;42(2):498–510.

13. Gladstone HB, Cohen JL. Adverse effects when injecting facial fillers. Semin Cutan Med Surg 2007; 26(1):34–9.

14. Chopra R, Graivier M, Fabi S, et al. A multi-center, open-label, prospective study of cannula injection of small-particle hyaluronic acid plus lidocaine (SPHAL) for lip augmentation. J Drugs Dermatol 2018;17(1):10–6.

15. Shah NS, Lazarus MC, Bugdodel R, et al. The effects of topical vitamin K on bruising after laser treatment. J Am Acad Dermatol 2002;47(2):241–4.

16. Fitzgerald R, Bertucci V, Sykes JM, et al. Adverse reactions to injectable fillers. Facial Plast Surg 2016; 32(5):532–55.

17. Signorini M, Liew S, Sundaram H, et al. Global aesthetics consensus group. Global aesthetics consensus: avoidance and management of complications from hyaluronic acid fillers-evidence- and opinion-based review and consensus recommendations. Plast Reconstr Surg 2016;137(6):961e–71e.

18. Van Dyke S, Hays GP, Caglia AE, et al. Severe acute local reactions to a hyaluronic acid-derived dermal filler. J Clin Aesthet Dermatol 2010;3(5):32–5.

19. Geisler D, Shumer S, Elson ML. Delayed hypersensitivity reaction to restylane. Cosmet Dermatol 2007;20(12):784–6.

20. Christensen LH. Host tissue interaction, fate, and risks of degradable and non-degradable gel fillers. Dermatol Surg 2009;35(Suppl 2):1612–9.

21. Sclafani AP, Fagien S. Treatment of injectable soft tissue filler complications. Dermatol Surg 2009;35: 1672–80.

22. Arron ST, Neuhaus IM. Persistent delayed-type hypersensitivity reaction to injectable non-animal-stabilized hyaluronic acid. J Cosmet Dermatol 2007;6(3):167–71.

23. Cassuto D, Marangoni O, De Santis G, et al. Advanced laser techniques for filler-induced complications. Dermatol Surg 2009;35(Suppl 2):1689–95.

24. Taylor SC, Burgess CM, Callender VD. Safety of nonanimal stabilized hyaluronic acid dermal fillers in patients with skin of color: a randomized, evaluator-blinded comparative trial. Dermatol Surg 2009;35(Suppl 2):1653–60.

25. Heath CR, Taylor SC. Fillers in the skin of color population. J Drugs Dermatol 2011;10(5):494–8.

26. DeLorenzi C. Complications of injectable fillers, part I. Aesthet Surg J 2013;33(4):561–75.

27. Hirsch RJ, Narurkar V, Carruthers J. Management of injected hyaluronic acid induced Tyndall effects. Lasers Surg Med 2006;38(3):202–4.

28. Douse-Dean T, Jacob CI. Fast and easy treatment for reduction of the Tyndall effect secondary to cosmetic use of hyaluronic acid. J Drugs Dermatol 2008;7(3):281–3.

29. Rousso JJ, Pitman MJ. Enterococcus faecalis complicating dermal filler injection: a case of virulent facial abscesses. Dermatol Surg 2010;36(10):1638–41.

30. Dayan SH, Arkins JP, Brindise R. Soft tissue fillers and biofilm. Facial Plast Surg 2011;27:23–8.

31. Ledon JA, Savas JA, Yang S, et al. Inflammatory nodules following soft tissue filler use: a review of causative agents, pathology and treatment options. Am J Clin Dermatol 2013;14:401–11.

32. Bjarnsholt T, Tolker-Nielsen T, Givskov M, et al. Detection of bacteria by fluorescence in situ hybridization in culture-negative soft tissue filler lesions. Dermatol Surg 2009;35(Suppl 2):1620–4.

33. Rzany B, DeLorenzi C. Understanding, avoiding, and managing severe filler complications. Plast Reconstr Surg 2015;136(5 Suppl):196S–203S.

34. Tohidnezhad M, Varoga D, Wruck CJ, et al. Platelets display potent antimicrobial activity and release human beta-defensin 2. Platelets 2012;23(3):217–23.

35. Albeiroti S, Ayasoufi K, Hill DR, et al. Platelet hyaluronidase-2: an enzyme that translocates to the surface upon activation to function in extracellular matrix degradation. Blood 2015;125(9):1460–9.

36. Lemperle G, Gauthier-Hazan N, Wolters M, et al. Foreign body granulomas after all injectable dermal fillers: part 1. Possible causes. Plast Reconstr Surg 2009;123(6):1842–63.

37. Lemperle G, Gauthier-Hazan N. Foreign body granulomas after all injectable dermal fillers: part 2. Treatment options. Plast Reconstr Surg 2009; 123(6):1864–73.

Tips to Avoid Complications Following Mohs Reconstruction

Andrew J. Kaufman, MD[a,b],*

KEYWORDS

- Facial reconstruction • Skin cancer • Mohs • Bilobed transposition flap
- Helical rim advancement flap • Island advancement flap • Forehead flap

KEY POINTS

- For most reconstructive procedures following Mohs or other skin cancer surgery, there are usually key elements in the design and implementation of the procedure that simplify and speed the technique, ensure good results, and avoid complications and bad results.
- The best practice is to learn and practice these elements to produce consistent good results and minimize the risk of bad or botched results.

INTRODUCTION

Once a "bad" result has occurred in reconstructive surgery, the old adage "the horse is already out of the barn" becomes more of a reality. Optimum cosmetic and functional results are generally easier the first time around before somebody has incised, undermined, cauterized, moved, and sutured tissue. Options for improvement can be somewhat limited at this point and are similar to techniques for improving bad results in cosmetic or other surgery. Trapdoor or pincushioning of a flap, like a hypertrophic scar, can be treated with monthly intralesional steroid injections and pressure or massage. Notching or depression of a scar can be improved with scar revision with or without a z-plasty or some other technique that "breaks up" a scar or changes secondary tension vectors. Hair transposed onto a recipient site can be surgically removed, epilated, or treated with a hair removal laser. One would really prefer to design and execute a repair in a fashion that avoids bad results. This is not as difficult as it may seem, as there are particular key elements in the design and performance of many repairs that help to avoid most suboptimal results. We discuss 4 very helpful repairs in facial reconstruction following skin cancer surgery and the tips to prevent poor outcomes.

BILOBED TRANSPOSITION FLAP

The bilobed transposition flap has been referred to as a "workhorse" flap for defects on the distal third of the nose, where there is less tissue mobility due to the thicker sebaceous nasal skin and the underlying cartilaginous support. The flap is useful for defects up to approximately 1.5 cm in diameter, and this author prefers to use this flap for non-midline defects (ie, defects on the nasal ala, lateral tip, and distal sidewall) (**Fig. 1**A). For midline defects, to maintain symmetry, the author prefers flaps that recruit tissue from both sides for the repair (eg, bilateral advancement flap for nasal dorsum and bilateral rotation flap for nasal tip).

Commercial or Financial Conflicts: The author has no commercial or financial conflicts of interest. The author has no outside funding sources.
[a] The Center for Dermatology Care, 267 West Hillcrest Drive, Thousand Oaks, CA 91360, USA; [b] Keck School of Medicine of University of Southern California, Los Angeles, CA, USA
* The Center for Dermatology Care, 267 West Hillcrest Drive, Thousand Oaks, CA 91360.

Facial Plast Surg Clin N Am 27 (2019) 571–579
https://doi.org/10.1016/j.fsc.2019.07.012
1064-7406/19/© 2019 Elsevier Inc. All rights reserved.

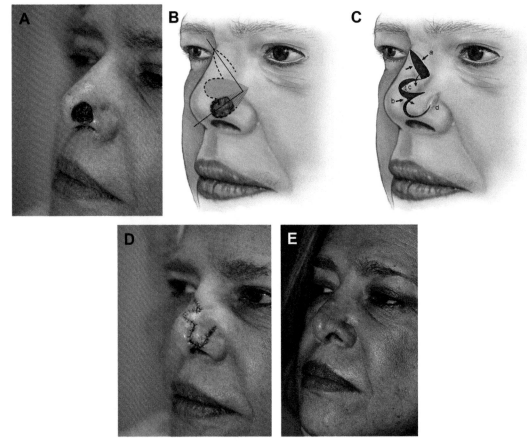

Fig. 1. (*A*) Surgical defect following Mohs surgery for basal cell carcinoma involving left nasal tip and soft triangle. (*B*) Design of bilobed transposition flap. Defect is anterior (ie, toward nasal midline) so lateral pedicle chosen. Tricone placed above alar crease (*hash-marked area*). Addition of first lobe of similar size and approximately 45° arc creates a heart-shaped or cordiform flap (*shaded area*). Addition of second lobe should be similar size and distance for a total or 90 to 100° arc. Second lobe should taper to 30 angle to facilitate closure. (*C*) After incision, wide undermining, confirmation of ease of transposition and hemostasis, first move is to close tertiary defect (a), followed by key suture placement in cleft between 2 lobes (b), followed by trimming of flaps if necessary (c) and finally excision of tricone (d), angling away from vascular pedicle if possible and avoiding interference with internal nasal valve. (*D*) Bilobed transposition flap sutured into place. (*E*) Short-term healed result at approximately 4 months.

The bilobed flap may be quite useful for defects on the distal third of the nose, but its transposition movement and complex design increase complications like trapdoor or pincushioning of the flap, as well as distortion of the nasal tip or ala. Through accurate and careful design and execution of the flap, the risk of these complications can be minimized.

The bilobed flap was originally described by Esser in 1918, but it was Zitelli's modification in 1989 that made it much more applicable and successful in nasal reconstruction.[1,2] Zitelli described 2 lobes of equal size approximately 45 to 50° apart and the excision of a tricone in the design of the flap. These insightful modifications made the flap more useful in creating aesthetic repairs for small to medium-sized defects. Still, the geometry of the flap and its transposition nature make it intimidating for many surgeons; however, by following several key concepts, it becomes a very straightforward and useful repair.

The first thing to understand is that the flap should be heart-shaped or cordiform in its design. The first and second lobes are the same diameter as the surgical defect. The distance from the surgical defect to the first lobe is the same as the distance from the first lobe to the second lobe. One should not reduce the size or arc of the first or second lobe. The first choice to make in planning the flap is whether the flap will have a medial pedicle or a lateral pedicle.[3] For surgical defects more anterior on the nose (ie, closer to the midline), a lateral pedicle is preferred; for defects more posterior (ie, closer to the nose-cheek junction), a medial pedicle works best. The point is to keep the flap located on one side of the nose, rather than crossing the mid portion of the nose if possible. Once the location of the pedicle is determined (ie, lateral vs medial), the tricone to be excised can be drawn out. The tricone should avoid crossing the alar crease and whenever possible sit at the junction of cosmetic nasal subunits. At this point in flap design, we have drawn out half of the "heart" (ie, surgical defect with attached tricone). The next step is to complete the heart-shaped flap, drawing in another same-sized lobe that is 45° from the tip of the tricone. The final step in design of the flap is to draw a second lobe, same size and same arc (ie, 45–50°) as the first one, but this lobe tapers to a 30° angle. This 30° angle will facilitate closure of the wound without development of a dog-ear or tricone (**Fig. 1**B). Flaps designed with disparate-sized lobes or angles increase the risk of depression or elevation of the alar rim or distortion of the nasal tip.

The flap is incised, and the author's preference is to leave excision of the tricone for the end of the procedure. The flap and surrounding area is undermined by blunt and sharp dissection in the submuscular plane on the nose (subcutaneous if undermining is extended onto the nose-cheek junction). After adequate undermining, transposition of the flap into the surgical defect is evaluated (in the author's experience surgeons occasionally do not undermine widely enough, especially around the site of the second lobe, which limits transposition of the flap). Once mobilization is complete and hemostasis is achieved by light spot electrocautery, the tertiary defect is closed. As a transposition flap, one of the key tenets in performing this repair is to close the tertiary defect first. In a rhombic transposition flap, the secondary defect is closed first; in a bilobed transposition flap, the tertiary defect (ie, site of the second lobe) is closed first. This one key process allows the flap to transpose over the intervening tissue and essentially "fall" into place. It is one of the reasons that properly performed transposition flaps can minimize secondary tension vectors around the surgical defect and are therefore quite useful near free margins or anatomic landmarks. So the first key point in transposing this flap is closure of the tertiary defect, and the second key point is to suture the cleft between the 2 lobes into its respective point at the surgical defect (**Fig. 1**C). This second key element maintains the properly designed geometry of the flap. By securing the cleft between the 2 lobes, the flap is placed in the exact proper anatomically neutral position. After that, it is only a matter of trimming the flaps slightly if too long, additional suturing, and

excision of the tricone, which one might angle slightly away from the pedicle and thus preserve maximum vascular supply. Buried sutures are used to close the rtertiary and secondary defects and to secure the first lobe into the surgical wound. These buried sutures around the first lobe within the surgical defect help secure the flap and may help decrease the chance of trapdooring or pincushioning. Final percutaneous sutures are running or simple interrupted, and a secure pressure bandage is applied for 24 hours (with nasal packing if pressure on the wound would cause collapse of the nasal ala during that 24 hours) (**Box 1**, **Fig. 1**D, E).

HELICAL RIM ADVANCEMENT FLAPS

One of the most useful and easy to perform reconstructions for defects limited to the helical rim is the helical rim advancement flap (**Fig. 2**A). First described by Antia and Buch in 1967,[4] a number of iterations of the flap have been proposed both in the scientific literature and lectures. Although some modifications may succeed and some may fail, there are a couple key elements in design and execution of this flap that avoid bad results like partial-thickness or full-thickness necrosis of the flap or notching of the helical rim.

First, in the design of the flap, the incision in the helical sulcus travels from the surgical defect all the way to the lobule.[5,6] The loose tissue is in the lobule. An advancement flap recruits tissue from where there is loose or redundant tissue and advances it into the surgical defect. A flap that stops along the helical rim without reaching the lobule is essentially stretching the flap or tissue because there is no significant redundant or loose tissue along the helical rim. So, first, the incision is

---

Box 1
Bilobed transposition flaps

Design bilobed transposition flap as heart-shaped (cordiform) with 2 similar-sized lobes 45 to 50° apart and include a tricone in the design.

Incision and undermining in submuscular plane on nose and subcutaneous on cheek. Make sure to undermine around the flap and surrounding tissue, including the tissue around the second lobe.

Close tertiary defect first and then close or secure the cleft between the 2 lobes.

Excise tricone, taking care to avoid cutting into the pedicle of the flap.

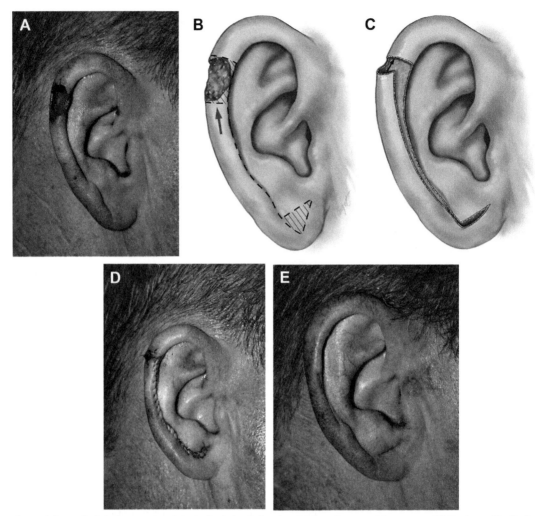

Fig. 2. (*A*) Surgical defect on the right helical rim following Mohs micrographic surgery. (*B*) Design of helical rim advancement flap. Surgical defect is extended to the helical sulcus if necessary (*hash-marked area on helical rim*). Incision lines at helical rim made perpendicular to skin surface to permit proper closure and eversion of incision line. Incision line follows helical sulcus all the way to the lobule where a tricone will be removed (*hash-marked triangle in lobule*). Incision through the sulcus and lobule are carried to the medial pinna but do not incise the cutaneous surface on the medial side. (*C*) Undermining widely on the medial side of the pinna to the postauricular sulcus helps to maintain a broad robust pedicle. After adequate undermining, the flap is advanced into the surgical defect and the tricone defect in the lobule closes. (*D*) Helical rim advancement flap sutured into place with 1 or 2 buried absorbable sutures at the helical rim. Secondary defect and flap sutured into place with buried absorbable sutures. Helical rim everted or hypereverted with nonabsorbable vertical mattress sutures. Tricone excised and closed on medial pinna and remaining cutaneous surface closed with running percutaneous suture. (*E*) Short-term healed result shows good reconstruction of helical rim.

carried all the way to the lobule. Within the lobule a tricone is excised (**Fig. 2**B). Removal of the tricone helps to release the flap and allows it to more easily advance into the surgical wound. But before the flap is advanced it must be undermined, and undermining is performed over the medial aspect of the pinna (ie, entire medial side of the pinna down to the post auricular sulcus). By making the incision through the helical sulcus down to *but not through* the skin on the medial aspect of

the pinna, a very broad, richly vascular pedicle is maintained (**Fig. 2**C). This is a better, safer technique than creating a tubed flap of just helical rim tissue with a more tenuous blood supply. After adequate undermining and hemostasis is completed, the flap is advanced into the helical rim surgical defect and sutured into place with buried absorbable suture (note: as an advancement flap, the defect, rather than the secondary defect, is closed *first*). After buried sutures have secured the flap within the surgical defect of the helical rim, the skin of the helical rim itself is approximated and everted with vertical mattress sutures. Taking care to hyper-evert the skin crossing the helical rim helps to prevent notching of the helical rim at a later time. The flap is secured along the helical sulcus and lobule with buried sutures and a running percutaneous suture. And finally, the tricone that developed on the medial aspect of the pinna after advancement of the flap is excised and the wound closed, thus preserving the broad vascular pedicle on the medial pinna (**Box 2**, **Fig. 2**D, E).

ISLAND ADVANCEMENT FLAPS

Island advancement flaps are useful for reconstruction in many regions, including the alar sill, the complex peninsula of tissue that separates the nose, lip, and cheek (**Fig. 3**A). Sometimes referred to as V-to-Y advancement flaps, subcutaneous pedicle flaps, or incorrectly as island pedicle flaps, these flaps may provide advantages over other options for repair in this region.[7–9] Rotation flap repairs may extend onto the cheek skin or cause upward lifting the ipsilateral oral commissure. Advancement or transposition flaps or side-to-side repairs in the region can risk blunting of the alar sill, which can be obvious because of a lack of symmetry when compared with the contralateral side.

Island advancement flaps lack a cutaneous attachment and therefore are more mobile than other random pattern flaps. The blood supply is based solely on the subcutaneous pedicle, and so proper design and handling of the tissue is of paramount importance. The flap works well for small to medium-sized defects in the alar sill, keeping the repair within one cosmetic subunit. Other benefits include placement of 2 of the triangular flap incision lines at subunit junctions, helping to hide the resultant scars, and avoidance of secondary tension vectors that could distort the lip or oral commissure.

In design of the island advancement flap, one long incision line follows the melolabial furrow and a second crosses the upper lip, gradually tapering to a point where it meets the first incision (**Fig. 3**B). By allowing a longer, more gradual taper to the flap, secondary tension vectors are minimized and the transition from cheek to upper lip appears more natural. After the triangular flap is incised, it is mobilized by careful blunt and sharp dissection, first at the leading edge (prevents bulldozing) and trailing edge (prevents tethering), and then along the sides. The key is a delicate balance between mobilization of the flap while maintaining a robust vascular pedicle. Undermining is complete when the leading edge of the flap can be secured into the surgical wound without significant tension. The flap is advanced into the surgical wound and secured with buried absorbable sutures. After this, the secondary defect and remaining flap edges are secured with similar sutures (**Fig. 3**C). The epidermis is approximated and everted with a running percutaneous nonabsorbable suture (**Fig. 3**D, E). As a result, one long side of the isosceles triangle is hidden within the melolabial furrow; the base side is hidden at the base of the nasal ala, and one of the base angles functions like a wedge, nicely reconstructing that missing peninsula of tissue between the nose, cheek, and lip (**Box 3**).

Box 3
Island advancement flaps

Island advancement flaps are useful for repairs of the alar sill because the repair is kept within 1 cosmetic unit, 2 of the incision lines are at the junction of cosmetic subunits and 1 of the base angles of the triangle may function well to replace the missing tissue that separates the nose, lip, and cheek.

The long sides of the triangle should be long and gradually taper to minimize secondary tension vectors and maintain a natural transition from cheek to lip.

Mobilization of the flap is a careful balancing act between undermining/mobilization and preservation of the vascular pedicle. Judicious blunt dissection and mindful evaluation of adequate mobilization help to meet these requirements.

As an advancement flap, first sutures are used to advance and secure the leading edge of the flap into the surgical defect. Subsequent sutures close the secondary defect that results after advancement of the flap.

Box 2
Helical rim advancement flaps

Incision of the helical rim advancement flap should follow the helical sulcus all the way to the lobule, where a tricone should be excised, facilitating advancement of the flap.

Incision through the helical sulcus should avoid incision through the skin on the medial pinna, thus preserving a broad vascular pedicle on the medial aspect of the pinna.

Vertical mattress sutures should be used crossing the helical rim to hyper-evert the helical rim closure and prevent notching.

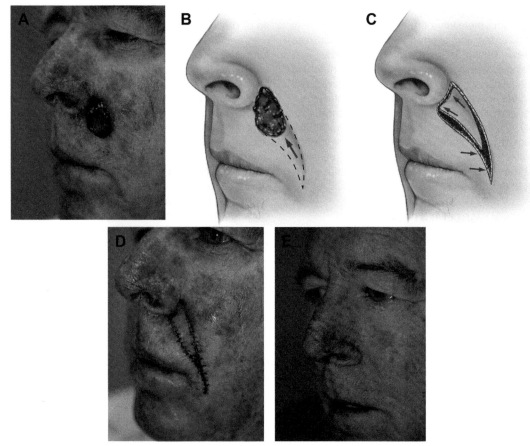

Fig. 3. (*A*) Post-Mohs surgical defect involving all of left alar sill. (*B*) Design of island advancement flap. Long, tapering triangular flap with one side following the melolabial furrow. (*C*) After incision of flap, proceed with careful blunt and sharp dissection to mobilize flap. Start by sharp dissection at leading edge (prevents bulldozing) and trailing edge (prevents tethering) and then continue on sides. Slow, gradual blunt dissection to balance mobilization of flap with preservation of vascular pedicle. Flap advanced into the surgical wound and sutured into place, creating a secondary defect that is subsequently closed (*horizontal arrows*). One base angle of the triangular flap functions as a reconstructive wedge of the peninsular-shaped alar sill between cheek, nose, and lip. (*D*) Island advancement flap sutured into place. (*E*) Short-term healed appearance demonstrates maintenance of alar sill and avoidance of blunting or obscuring that well-defined region.

PARAMEDIAN FOREHEAD FLAP

One of the earliest forms of nasal reconstruction, the forehead flap, dates to the sixth century BC, when it was first described in an ancient Sanskrit text on medicine and surgery.[10] Subsequently, the text and the procedure were brought to Sicily and then ultimately reached an English-language audience when it was first described in a Letter to the Editor in *Gentleman's Magazine* in 1794.[11] More than 200 years after it reached an English audience, the procedure is quite different from what was originally described in India more than 2000 years ago, but remains a highly useful reconstructive method for large or complex nasal defects (**Fig. 4**A).[12] Still, there are key principles in design and execution that must be followed to avoid complications with this reliable repair.

The paramedian forehead flap is an axial pattern flap, based on the supratrochlear artery and other nearby contributory vessels.[13] Design of the flap is no longer "midline," but rather "paramedian," suggesting the flap is adjacent to the midline on one side or the other. The author's preference is to select the side ipsilateral to the surgical defect. An ipsilateral flap might twist a greater arc but can reach a greater distance than a contralateral flap. In a proper forehead flap, the extra twisting does not impact the flap's

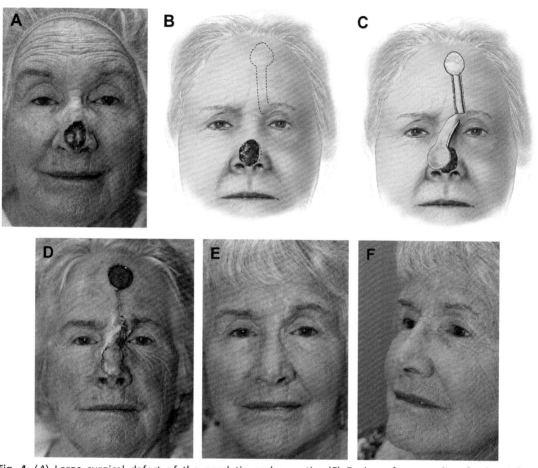

Fig. 4. (*A*) Large surgical defect of the nasal tip and supratip. (*B*) Design of paramedian forehead flap. Defect slightly enlarged in areas so incision lines would fall at the junction of cosmetic subunits (*dashed lines on nasal tip and supratip*). Template taken and placed just below hairline. Pedicle measures between 1.2 and 1.5 cm and is centered over the glabellar furrow. Pedicle goes from glabellar furrow to base of template. A 4 × 4 gauze or ruler may be used to measure and confirm that flap will reach surgical defect without significant tension. If necessary, the medial incision may be carried out just below the orbital rim, taking care to avoid trauma to nearby blood vessels (see *C* also). (*C*) Flap is incised into the very superficial subcutaneous fat beneath the template, which permits more rapid and improved healing of donor site by second intention healing. When the incision approaches the narrow pedicle it should dive down through the subcutaneous fat and frontalis muscle to the periosteum and remain in this plane for the remainder of the mobilization proximally. The supratrochlear artery is sandwiched between the corrugator and frontalis muscles as it crosses the orbital rim, so the vascular supply is protected if one remains in the proper plane and avoids trauma to nearby blood vessels. (*D*) Paramedian forehead flap sutured into place. Exposed area of pedicle carefully wrapped with petrolatum/bismuth-impregnated gauze, which helps keep the pedicle moist and avoids excessive drainage. Secondary defect on superior forehead to superficial subcutaneous tissue allowed to heal by second intention healing (wound kept moist and covered to facilitate healing). (*E*) Healed result at 4 months shows fairly well healed result. There is good color, texture, and thickness to the reconstructed area. Incision lines or scars could be improved by scarabrasion or laser resurfacing, but patient was quite pleased with result and refused further touch up. (*F*) Oblique view of healed result shows good cosmetic and functional outcome.

viability; however, difficulty in reaching the surgical defect without significant tension can impact blood flow. So for defects on the right side of the nose, the flap would be based on the right side of the forehead. For midline nasal surgical defects, either side of the forehead may be used,

and if the forehead has significant scarring on one side, the contralateral side is probably more reliable.

The first step in the design of the flap is to create a template of the surgical defect. If necessary, the surgical defect should be enlarged or extended so that the incision lines will be at the junction of cosmetic subunits, and therefore, the resultant scars will be less noticeable. Any enlargement of the defect should be factored into the resulting template. The author prefers the use of a nonadherent bandage (eg, Telfa) to create the template, and this is then placed on the forehead just inferior to the frontal hairline. One of the most common, yet easily avoidable, complications is the transfer of permanent, terminal hairs from the frontal scalp to the surgical wound on the nose. Epilation, laser hair removal, and even surgical excision of hair bulbs work inconsistently in some of these cases. There are much easier ways to lengthen the reach of the flap without extending into the frontal scalp. One option would be to move the template to the midforehead or cross to the contralateral superior forehead while keeping the pedicle on the ipsilateral side. After all, the rich vascular plexus on the forehead would still support this longer angled flap so long as the blood supply is carefully preserved in creation of the flap. Another option routinely performed to lengthen the flap reach is to carefully extend the medial incision to just below the orbital rim. To succeed in this approach, we need to understand proper design of the paramedian forehead flap and understand the anatomy involved.

The supratrochlear artery, the mainstay of the flap pedicle, crosses the orbital rim deep to the glabellar furrow, sandwiched between the corrugator and frontalis muscles. The artery travels superiorly and in the mid forehead passes through the frontalis muscle and continues upward in the subcutaneous tissue. As a result, the pedicle of the flap should be between 1.2 and 1.5 cm in width, with the center over the glabellar furrow (or perhaps favoring just to the medial aspect of the furrow by approximately 0.2 cm). The pedicle is drawn out at this same width until it reaches the outline of the surgical defect template on the superior forehead inferior to the hairline (**Fig. 4**B).

The flap is incised to the superficial subcutaneous fat at the site of the template. Most of the time a very small amount of fat is necessary to reconstruct the distal third of the nose, and too much fat frequently necessitates a debulking procedure at the time of the division and inset or another later time. The exception might be in smokers, in which case a slightly greater amount of fat may be left on the distal aspect of the flap. Once the portion of the flap that will cover the nasal defect is incised and the incision approaches the narrower pedicle, the incision dives down to the periosteum (ie, deep to the frontalis muscle) and stays there. From this point

inferiorly, the incision and blunt dissection continue along the periosteum and therefore the supratrochlear artery is protected within the pedicle. If additional flap length or reach is necessary, careful undermining and careful extension of the medial incision can be extended just below the orbital rim, taking care to avoid trauma to blood vessels.

After the flap has been incised, adequate reach of the flap to the surgical defect confirmed, and careful hemostasis achieved, the secondary defect (ie, donor site on the forehead) can be closed (**Fig. 4**C). The length of the pedicle is closed with buried absorbable sutures. Because of the superficial or shallow nature of the wound on the superior forehead, this aspect of the donor site may be allowed to heal by second intention healing with very good results. As a result, no skin grafts or flaps or undo-pressure to close the secondary defect is needed. The paramedian forehead flap is transposed and sutured into the surgical defect with minimal or no tension using buried and percutaneous sutures. The author prefers to carefully wrap a petrolatum/bismuth-impregnated gauze around the open pedicle, holding it in place with several small superficial sutures and avoiding ligation of accessory blood vessels (**Fig. 4**D). A pressure bandage is applied for 24 hours to the donor and recipient sites but avoids pressure to the pedicle. Sutures are removed as routine at 7 days, and the pedicle is divided and inset 3

Box 4
Paramedian forehead flaps

The paramedian forehead flap is usually designed so that the pedicle is ipsilateral to the surgical defect unless scarring or some other factor would favor a contralateral pedicle.

Pedicle is 1.2 to 1.5 cm in width and centered over the glabellar furrow or centered just 1 to 2 mm medial to the furrow.

Pedicle travels upward with the same width until it reaches the template, located just inferior to the frontal hairline.

Incision of the flap is limited to the superficial subcutaneous fat beneath the templated area, which will cover the surgical defect. When the incision approaches the narrower pedicle, the incision dives deep to the periosteum and stays there as it continues inferiorly.

If necessary to increase reach of the flap, the medial incision can be extended carefully a small amount just beyond the orbital rim, taking care to avoid damage to nearby vessels.

to 4 weeks after the first surgery. Second intention healing with proper wound care instructions is usually almost complete at the time of division and inset (**Box 4, Fig. 4**E, F)

SUMMARY

In conclusion, for most reconstructive procedures following Mohs or other skin cancer surgery, there are usually key elements in the design and implementation of the procedure that simplify and speed the technique, ensure good results, and avoid complications and bad results. The best practice is to learn and practice these elements and produce consistent good results and minimize the risk of bad or botched results.

REFERENCES

1. Esser JFS. Gestielte lokale nasenplastik mit zweizipfligem lappen, deckung des sekundaren defektes vom ersten zifel durch den zweiten. Dtsch Zschr Chir 1918;143:385–90.
2. Zitelli JA. The bilobed flap for nasal reconstruction. Arch Dermatol 1989;125:957–9.
3. Kaufman AJ. Nasal sidewall and supratip: bilobed transposition flap, lateral pedicle. In: Practical facial reconstruction: theory and practice. Philadelphia: Wolters Kluwer; 2017. p. 111–20.
4. Antia NH, Buch VI. Chrondrocutaneous advancement flap for the marginal defect of the ear. Plast Reconstr Surg 1967;39:472–7.
5. Kaufman AJ. Helical rim advancement flaps for reconstruction. Dermatol Surg 2008;34:1229–32.
6. Kaufman AJ. Helical rim: helical rim advancement flap. In: Practical facial reconstruction: theory and practice. Philadelphia: Wolters Kluwer; 2017. p. 230–8.
7. Rustad TJ, Hartshorn DO, Clevens RA, et al. The subcutaneous pedicle flap in melolabial reconstruction. Arch Otolaryngol Head Neck Surg 1998;124:1163–6.
8. Chapman JT, Mellette JR Jr. Perioral reconstruction. In: Rohrer TE, Cook JL, Nguyen TH, et al, editors. Flaps and grafts in dermatologic surgery. Philadelphia: Saunders Elsevier; 2007. p. 217–34.
9. Kaufman AJ. Alar sill: island advancement flap. In: Practical facial reconstruction: theory and practice. Philadelphia: Wolters Kluwer; 2017. p. 174–9.
10. Burget GC, Menick FJ. Aesthetic reconstruction of the nose. St Louis (MO): Mosby; 1994.
11. BL. The gentleman's magazine and historical chronicle, vol. 64, 1794. p. 891–2.
12. Burget GC, Menick FJ. The paramedian forehead flap. In: Aesthetic reconstruction of the nose. St Louis (MO): Mosby; 1994. p. 57–61.
13. Shumrick KA, Smith TL. The anatomical basis for the design of forehead flaps in nasal reconstruction. Arch Otolaryngol Head Neck Surg 1992;118:373–9.

Moving?

Make sure your subscription moves with you!

To notify us of your new address, find your **Clinics Account Number** (located on your mailing label above your name), and contact customer service at:

Email: journalscustomerservice-usa@elsevier.com

800-654-2452 (subscribers in the U.S. & Canada)
314-447-8871 (subscribers outside of the U.S. & Canada)

Fax number: 314-447-8029

Elsevier Health Sciences Division
Subscription Customer Service
3251 Riverport Lane
Maryland Heights, MO 63043

*To ensure uninterrupted delivery of your subscription, please notify us at least 4 weeks in advance of move.

Printed and bound by CPI Group (UK) Ltd, Croydon, CR0 4YY

08/05/2025

01864747-0016